# Make Yourself More Attractive

**Dr. Wade**

# Contents

# Summary

Unleash Your Inner Radiance: A Guide to Becoming More Attractive is a transformative book that empowers readers to increase their personal attractiveness by focusing on inner transformation and self-acceptance. With practical advice and insightful advice, this book takes readers on a journey of self-discovery, encouraging them to embrace their unique qualities and inspire confidence.

The book challenges conventional beauty standards and emphasizes the importance of self-love and acceptance. Encourage readers to forego external verification and instead develop a positive attitude and strong self-esteem. By embracing their authentic selves, readers can unleash their true attraction.

Physical well-being is also covered and the book offers advice on healthy lifestyles, self-care practices and personal style. Emphasize the importance of taking care of your body, choosing clothing that reflects your individual characteristics, and cultivating a personal style that reflects your true self. By physically taking care of themselves, readers can enhance their natural beauty and increase their self-esteem.

In addition, the book explores the power of effective communication and meaningful connections. It explores the importance of active listening, positive body language and storytelling to connect with others. By developing strong communication skills, readers can increase their appeal and make a lasting impression.

Throughout the book, readers are encouraged to show compassion for themselves and to refrain from judgment. Emphasize the importance of valuing yourself and recognizing your innate worth. By embracing self-love, readers can inspire confidence and self-confidence, which ultimately contributes to their overall attractiveness.

"Unleash Your Inner Glory: A Guide to Becoming More Attractive" celebrates a journey of self-discovery and personal development. It guides readers to embrace their unique qualities, nurture their physical wellbeing, and develop a positive attitude. By unleashing their inner brilliance and embodying their authentic selves, readers can increase their appeal in an authentic and uplifting way.

# Preface

Welcome to Unleash Your Inner Glow: A Journey to Personal Attractiveness. In a world where standards of beauty are often determined by external factors, this book aims to bring attention back to the power of inner transformation. It is a guide to help you discover and embrace your unique qualities, increasing your attractiveness from within.

We live in a society that attaches great importance to appearances. Advertising, social media, and cultural norms often determine what is considered attractive. However, the real appeal goes beyond the aesthetics of the surface. It's about harnessing your individuality, inspiring confidence, and embodying the essence of your authentic self.

This book is not about conforming to societal ideals or obtaining outside approval. Instead, it is a journey of self-discovery, self-acceptance, and self-love. It is an invitation to explore the depths of your being and discover the beauty within you.

Throughout the pages of this book you will find practical advice, inspirational stories, and transformational exercises that will lead you to a more attractive version of yourself. But let's be clear: the goal isn't to change who you are. Rather, it's about embracing your unique qualities and honing them in ways that give you a sense of confidence and strength.

We will discuss the various aspects of personal attractiveness, beginning with the importance of cultivating a positive attitude. Your thoughts and beliefs shape your reality, so we explore techniques for cultivating self-love, positive affirmations, and a growth mindset.

Physical well-being is also a key factor in attractiveness. We examine the role of diet, exercise and self-care in improving your physical appearance. It should be emphasized that it is not about conforming to society's standards of beauty, but rather about nourishing and caring for the body in a way that suits individual needs.

Personal style and grooming are powerful tools for self-expression and attractiveness. We delve into the art of dressing for your body type, discovering your unique style and making treatment decisions that highlight your natural features.

But attractiveness isn't just about the physical aspect. We will also explore the transformative power of intrinsic qualities. Kindness, empathy, and gratitude are qualities that can take your attractiveness to a new level.

In this journey of personal attraction, it is important to realize that there will be ups and downs. Self-improvement is not linear and each journey is unique. But remember, the most attractive version of yourself is the one that is authentic and true to who you are.

I hope this book will be a trusted companion on your journey to unleashing your inner brilliance. I allow you to embrace your unique qualities, cultivate self-love, and unleash confidence and beauty from within. Remember that you are already attractive in your own way and this journey is about discovering and strengthening that innate attraction.

This is the release of your inner glow and the beginning of a transformative journey toward self-attractiveness.

# Prologue

In a world full of pictures of painted perfection and social pressure to conform, it is easy to feel overwhelmed and insecure about your own attractiveness. We often crave outside approval as we try to live up to society's standards of beauty. But what if the true appeal is not in the eyes of others, but in us?

Welcome to make you more attractive: unleash your inner glow. In this book we embark on a transformative journey that explores the depths of self-attraction and enables you to unleash your inner brilliance.

Attractiveness is not a fixed term that is defined solely by outward appearance. It is a multidimensional quality that includes our thoughts, our emotions, our actions and the energy we give off. True attractiveness comes from self-love, authenticity, and confidence. It's about embracing and appreciating our unique qualities, not fitting into a pattern.

This journey begins with self-reflection and introspection. We need to remove layers of social conditioning, shed the weight of insecurity, and reconnect with our authentic selves. It forces us to confront the limiting beliefs that have been holding us back and adopt a mindset of growth and self-acceptance.

In this book you will discover practical strategies and exercises to increase your attractiveness holistically. We explore the power of self-care, from supporting your physical wellbeing through exercise and diet, to developing a skincare routine that honors and enhances your natural beauty. But beyond the physical, we delve into the importance of emotional well-being, nurturing positive relationships, and developing an attitude of gratitude and self-compassion.

Personal style and self-expression are critical to attractiveness. We explore how you can express your individuality through fashion, hairstyling and the art of authentic presentation. By matching your outside to your inside, you exude confidence and attraction.

Communication skills also play an important role in attractiveness. We will explore the power of effective communication, active listening and non-verbal cues. When you learn to truly connect with others and form meaningful relationships, you increase your attractiveness and enrich your life.

But perhaps the most important aspect of this journey is the awareness that true attractiveness starts from within. It's about recognizing your worth, utilizing your strengths, and embracing the uniqueness that sets you apart. By cultivating self-love and self-acceptance, you radiate a radiant energy that draws others to you.

As we embark on this transformative journey together, remember that attractiveness is not a goal, but an ongoing process of self-development and self-discovery. Accept challenges, celebrate victories, and be patient with yourself while you do it.
So let's begin this journey of self-discovery and self-development. We unleash the power of our inner radiance and become the most attractive version of ourselves. The power is within you and this book will serve as your guide on this transformational journey.

Are you ready to become more attractive? Let's embark on this adventure together.

# Forward

In today's society, the pursuit of attractiveness has become an essential part of our lives. We are bombarded with images of flawless people, glamorous lifestyles and unattainable standards of beauty. The pressure to conform and live up to these ideals can leave us feeling inadequate and disconnected from our worth.

This is why Make Yourself More Attractive: Unleash Your Inner Beauty is such a timely and indispensable book. It challenges the notion that attractiveness is all about appearances and offers a refreshing perspective that allows people to cultivate their inner radiance.

Authentic attractiveness is not limited to a specific figure, perfect skin or fashionable clothes. It is a profound and transformative energy that radiates from within. It is about embracing and strengthening our unique qualities, promoting our physical and emotional well-being and developing a positive attitude.

In this book you embark on a journey of self-discovery and self-development. You will learn the power of self-acceptance and self-love as building blocks of attractiveness. By breaking free from comparison and peer pressure, you will find the freedom to embrace your true self and appreciate the beauty that is within you.

Through hands-on practice, inspirational stories and expert advice, you'll learn how to take care of your physical well-being and bring out your natural beauty. From establishing a self-care routine to understanding the importance of diet and exercise, you'll discover how these practices contribute to your overall attractiveness. The book also looks at the importance of personal style, emphasizing the importance of expressing yourself and dressing in a way that reflects one's identity. You will learn to match your outside to your inside, creating a sense of harmony and self-confidence.

Additionally, this book affirms the power of effective communication and making meaningful connections. You will learn strategies for developing strong interpersonal skills, active listening, and building authentic relationships. By mastering the art of connection, you increase your attractiveness and leave lasting impressions.

Make You More Attractive is not a quick guide or recipe for compliance. It is a roadmap to self-discovery, self-acceptance and self-development. It recognizes that attractiveness is a personal and subjective journey and that the destination is unique to each person.

As you embark on this transformational journey, I encourage you to approach it with an open mind and an open heart. Challenge yourself and allow yourself to be sensitive. Remember that true attractiveness isn't about getting approval from others, it's about embracing your authentic self and radiating that energy into the world.

I admire you for taking the first step in unleashing your inner beauty. By investing in yourself and starting this journey, you are already well on your way to becoming a more attractive and powerful person.

Let this book be your guide, offering ideas, inspiration and practical tools to unleash your inner brilliance. I wish you a transformative and rewarding journey in discovering and embracing your unique charm.

# Chapter No. 1

# Embracing Your Authentic Self

## Intro:

In a world that often places an emphasis on conformism and social norms, it's easy to lose touch with our true selves. This chapter invites you on a transformative journey of self-discovery and self-acceptance as we explore the power to embrace your authentic self. By letting go of outside expectations and accepting your uniqueness, you can release the essence of your attractiveness.

## Recognizing the Importance of Authenticity:

Here we explore why accepting your authentic self is critical to personal growth and attractiveness. We explore how social pressure, media influence and comparison can cause us to detach from our true identity. When you understand the implications of living authentically, you can begin to prioritize self-discovery and self-expression.

## Introspection and Self-Awareness:

Introspection is an essential tool in understanding who we really are. In this section, we guide you through self-reflection exercises and tips to help you better understand your values, passions, strengths, and weaknesses. By becoming more self-aware, you can align your actions with your authentic self and make choices that reflect your true desires and aspirations.

## Embrace Your Uniqueness:

We all have unique qualities that make us unique. This chapter discusses the importance of embracing your individuality and celebrating what makes you different from others. We discuss how comparisons can affect self-acceptance and offer strategies for boosting self-confidence and appreciating your unique qualities. By using your quirks, talents, and perspectives, you can shine with your authentic self-expression and attract others.

## Overcoming the Fear of Judgment:

Fear of judgment can prevent us from fully embracing our authentic selves. In this section, we share practical techniques and mindsets to help you overcome your fear of being judged by others. By challenging self-limiting beliefs and reformulating negative thoughts, you can develop the courage to be true to yourself and speak in your authentic voice without fear.

## Aligning Actions with Values:

Living by core values is essential to maintaining authenticity. In this chapter you will learn how to identify your values and align your actions with them. We discuss the importance of integrity and how living your values can lead to meaning and fulfillment. By making choices that are consistent with your true self, you exude a genuine sense of authenticity and attract others who appreciate your true nature.

## Self-Expression:

Self-expression is an effective way to present your authentic self to the world. We explore different forms of self-expression such as art, writing, fashion and hobbies and encourage you to find creative ways that allow you to express yourself authentically. Whether it's about your personal style, your artistic endeavors, or sharing your thoughts and ideas, self-expression is a liberating act that brings out your true self.

## Embrace growth and advancement:

Authenticity does not end; it evolves as we grow and learn. This chapter emphasizes the importance of personal development and openness to change. Discussing the concept of using discomfort as a catalyst for personal transformation, we encourage you to have new experiences, learn from your mistakes, and embrace new perspectives. By constantly evolving and embracing new opportunities, you can stay in touch with your authentic self and draw positive development into your life.

## Conclusion:

Coming to terms with your authentic self is a lifelong journey that requires self-reflection, self-acceptance and a willingness to be vulnerable. By rejecting social expectations, accepting your uniqueness, and aligning your actions with your values, you can radiate a compelling energy that draws others to your authentic self. In the following chapters we will look at the different aspects of self-attractiveness, all of which are based on the acceptance of one's authentic self. Remember that true attractiveness comes from within and by accepting yourself you can reach your full potential and live a truly fulfilling life.

# Chapter No. 2

# The Power of Inner Confidence

# Introduction:

Confidence is a magnetic quality that radiates from within and draws others to us. In this chapter, we delve into the transformative power of cultivating inner confidence and explore how it contributes to our overall attraction. By developing a strong sense of self and confidence in our abilities, we can face life with balance, authenticity and resilience.

# Understanding Inner Confidence:

Confidence goes beyond surface appearances and outward affirmation. It springs from a deep sense of self-worth and self-acceptance. In this section we explore the roots of inner trust and how it lays the foundation for personal growth and attractiveness. By understanding the true nature of inner trust, we can begin the journey of cultivating it within ourselves.

# Self-Acceptance:

Self-acceptance is a fundamental aspect of inner confidence. We discuss the importance of considering all aspects of ourselves, including our strengths, weaknesses, and imperfections. By cultivating self-acceptance, we free ourselves from the need for external validation and embrace our authentic selves. This acceptance allows us to go through life with grace and authenticity and to exude a genuine sense of confidence.

# Overcoming Insecurity and Limiting Beliefs:

Insecurity and limiting beliefs can undermine our self-esteem and prevent us from reaching our full potential. In this section we look at practical strategies for recognizing and challenging these negative thought patterns. By realigning our minds, adopting a growth mentality, and replacing self-doubt with confidence, we can overcome the obstacles that hamper our sense of self and lay a solid foundation for personal growth.

# Set Realistic Goals and Celebrate Success:

Goal setting plays a key role in building self-confidence. We engage in the process of setting realistic and achievable goals in line with our values and aspirations. By breaking bigger goals down into smaller steps, we create a sense of progress and accomplishment. Celebrating every achievement along the way boosts our confidence and fuels our motivation to achieve more.

# Developing Competence and Mastering Skills:

Competence creates self-confidence. This chapter emphasizes the importance of continuous learning, developing skills, and honing our talents. By investing in personal and professional development, we expand our knowledge base and experience, which in turn increases our confidence in our abilities. By developing skills in areas that align with our passions and interests, we naturally develop a sense of confidence and self-control.

## Maintain A Positive Internal Dialogue:

Our internal conversation has a major impact on our self-confidence. Here we explore techniques for cultivating positive self-talk and encouraging supportive thoughts. By practicing self-compassion, challenging negative self-talk and replacing it with affirming and empowering affirmations, we can shift our mindset toward trust. This positive internal dialogue strengthens our self-confidence and enables us to master challenges with resilience.

## Embracing and Burdening Failure:

 Failure is an inevitable part of life, but it doesn't define us. This section emphasizes the importance of accepting failure as an opportunity to grow and learn. By seeing failure as a step to success, we foster resilience and develop a fearless attitude in the face of challenges. When we accept failure as a natural part of the learning process, we increase our confidence and prepare ourselves to emerge stronger.

## Boosting Self-Confidence:

Confidence in your own body is an essential part of self-confidence. We explore strategies for developing body positive image, self-care and the practice of self-love. By maintaining a healthy relationship with our bodies and embracing our unique physical attributes, we boost our confidence and radiate magnetic energy that attracts others.

## Summary:

Inner trust is a transformative quality that has the power to improve all aspects of our lives. By accepting ourselves, confronting self-doubt, setting achievable goals, developing skills, encouraging positive self-talk, being resilient to setbacks, and cultivating self-confidence, we can develop strong self-confidence. By embodying this confidence, we create an compelling aura of confidence that draws others in and opens the door to opportunity. Over the next chapters we will continue to explore the elements that make us attractive, all rooted in the power of inner trust.

# Chapter No. 3

# Cultivating Self-Love and Self-Acceptance

## Introduction:

Self-love and self-acceptance are fundamental aspects of self-confidence and personal development. In this chapter we will explore the transformative power of developing a deep sense of self-love and acceptance. By accepting our true selves, accepting our strengths and weaknesses, and nurturing a compassionate relationship with ourselves, we can develop a deep level of self-love and self-acceptance that radiates outward and increases our attraction.

## Embrace Authenticity:

Authenticity is at the heart of self-love and self-acceptance. It's about embracing and expressing our true selves, free from the constraints of societal expectations and external validation. When we embrace our authentic selves, we step into the world with confidence and vulnerability. By respecting our values, passions and beliefs and living in harmony with our true nature, we develop a deep sense of self-love and acceptance. This authenticity allows us to make real connections and build relationships based on mutual respect and understanding.

## Self-Care:

Self-care is a fundamental aspect of self-love and self-acceptance. It is about prioritizing our physical, emotional and spiritual well-being. Regular self-care practices such as exercise, feeding our bodies nutrient-rich foods, getting enough rest, and activities that bring us joy and relaxation foster a deep sense of love, cleanliness, and caring. When taking care of ourselves is our priority, we are sending ourselves a powerful message that we deserve love and attention. By taking care of ourselves, we recharge our batteries and create a strong foundation for self-love and acceptance.

## Celebrating Strengths and Achievements:

Recognizing and celebrating our strengths and achievements is a powerful way to encourage self-love and self-acceptance. Each of us has unique talents, skills and traits that make us unique. By recognizing and using our strengths, we build a positive self-image and strengthen our self-confidence. It's important to take the time to celebrate our successes, no matter how small. This act of celebration builds our confidence and encourages us to keep growing and pursuing our goals with enthusiasm and confidence.

## Acceptance of Imperfections and Development:

Self-acceptance is about accepting one's imperfections and seeing them as opportunities for growth and learning. We are all imperfect and that is what makes us human. Accepting our imperfections means fully accepting yourself, your flaws and everything. By accepting our weaknesses, we can develop compassion for ourselves and for others. By recognizing that mistakes are a natural part of life, we free ourselves from the need for perfection and allow ourselves to grow and evolve. This acceptance of our shortcomings allows us to develop a deep sense of self-love and acceptance.

## Getting Rid of Self-Judgment:

 Self-judgment can be a significant impediment to self-esteem and self-acceptance. The critical voice within us can erode our self-esteem and perpetuate feelings of inadequacy. To cultivate self-esteem, we must practice self-compassion and replace self-judgment with self-kindness. This includes challenging negative self-talk, reformulating our thoughts, and treating ourselves with the same care and understanding that we treat others. When we let go of our self-esteem, we create a nurturing inner environment that supports our self-love and acceptance.

## Setting Boundaries and Prioritizing Needs:

Setting healthy boundaries is essential to self-love and self-acceptance. This includes acknowledging our needs, being assertive, and setting boundaries that honor our well-being. When we set boundaries, we create a safe space in which to prioritize our needs, protect our energy, and develop self-esteem. This act of self-care shows us and others that we value and respect ourselves. This allows us to build healthier relationships and interactions based on mutual respect and understanding.

## Cultivating Gratitude:

Gratitude is a powerful practice that deepens our sense of self-love and appreciation for life. By cultivating an attitude of gratitude, we focus on the positive aspects of ourselves and our experiences. When we express gratitude for our strengths, achievements, and even challenges, we can see ourselves in a more positive light. Gratitude opens our hearts to self-love and acceptance, and reminds us of the abundance and blessings all around us. It helps us to develop a deeper sense of self-worth and promotes a positive attitude towards life.

## Surround Yourself With Positive Influencers:

The people we surround ourselves with have a major impact on how we perceive ourselves and how we feel about ourselves. To foster self-love and self-acceptance, you must choose supportive and positive relationships. Surrounding ourselves with people who uplift, inspire, and celebrate creates an environment that boosts our self-esteem and acceptance. When we surround ourselves with love and positivity, we strengthen our belief that we deserve love and develop a deep sense of self-worth. These positive influences can include friends, family, mentors, and even online communities that share our values and support our personal growth.

## Conclusion:

Cultivating self-love and self-acceptance is a transformative journey that increases our inner confidence and attractiveness. By accepting our authenticity, taking care of ourselves, celebrating our strengths, accepting our imperfections, letting go of self-criticism, setting boundaries, cultivating gratitude, and surrounding ourselves with positive influences, we nourish our souls and develop a deep sense of love and acceptance for ourselves.

By radiating self-love and self-acceptance, we attract others who appreciate us for who we really are, make meaningful connections, and improve our overall well-being. Embracing self-love is not only a gift to ourselves, but also a gift to the world because we inspire others to embark on their own journey of self-acceptance and self-love.

# Chapter No. 4

# Nurturing Your Physical Well-Being

## Introduction:

In this chapter, we will examine the importance of physical well-being as a fundamental aspect of overall attractiveness and well-being. Your physical health plays a big role in how you feel and how others see you. By focusing on self-care practices that promote physical wellness, you can increase your attractiveness and create a positive connection with your body.

## Prioritize Regular Exercise:

Regular exercise is essential to maintaining a healthy body and mind. Physical activity not only improves fitness, but also improves mood, gives energy and reduces stress. Find an exercise you enjoy, whether it's jogging, dancing, swimming, or yoga, and incorporate it into your routine on a regular basis. Not only does this help maintain a toned, athletic figure, but it also promotes your overall well-being and boosts your confidence.

## Nourish your body with a healthy diet:

A balanced, nutritious diet is essential to maintaining physical well-being. Fueling your body with nutrient-dense foods gives you the energy and vitality you need to thrive. Include a variety of fruits, vegetables, whole grains, lean proteins, and healthy fats in your meals. Keep yourself well hydrated by drinking enough water throughout the day. By nourishing your body with the right foods, you can improve your complexion, maintain a healthy weight, and promote optimal body function.

## Adequate Rest and Sleep:

Adequate rest and sleep are essential for the regeneration of body and mind. Lack of sleep can negatively impact your appearance, mood, and overall well-being. Try to get a good night's sleep for 7 to 9 hours each night to give your body time to rest and re-energize. Establish a relaxed bedtime routine and create a comfortable sleeping environment to promote restful sleep. When you prioritize rest and sleep, not only do you improve your physical attractiveness, but you also improve cognition, mood, and overall health.

## Practicing Skin Care and Grooming:

Taking care of your skin and adopting good skin care habits can make a significant contribution to your physical appearance and self-confidence. Develop a skincare routine that includes cleansing, exfoliating, hydrating, and sunscreen. Take care of your hair, nails and personal hygiene to present yourself neatly. These simple self-care practices will not only improve your physical appearance but also boost your self-confidence.

## Maintaining Good Posture and Body Language:

Your posture and body language play a large role in how others perceive you and how you feel. Stand tall with your shoulders back and head up to show your confidence and attractiveness. Watch your body language and use open, friendly gestures to express friendliness and helpfulness. By maintaining good posture and positive body language, you exude confidence and appear more attractive to others.

## Prioritize stress management and relaxation:

Chronic stress can affect your physical well-being and appearance. To maintain your attractiveness and overall health, it's important to manage stress and focus on relaxation. Incorporate stress management techniques such as meditation, breathing exercises, and activities that bring joy and relaxation. By managing stress effectively, you can prevent its negative effects, including premature aging and weight gain.

## Embrace Movement and Physical Expression:

Movement and physical expression are key to promoting physical well-being and increasing attractiveness. Engage in activities that allow you to express yourself physically, such as dancing, yoga, or exercising. As well as improving your fitness, these classes will give you confidence and help you connect with your body on a deeper level.

## Incorporating Mind-Body Exercises:

In addition to exercising, incorporating mind-body exercises into your routine can make a significant contribution to your physical well-being. Activities like yoga, tai chi, and qigong not only promote flexibility and strength, but also help you connect with your body and develop a sense of inner peace. These exercises combine movement, breathwork, and mindfulness to release tension, improve posture, and increase body awareness. By incorporating mind-body practices into your life, you can holistically promote your physical well-being and support both body and mind.

## Regular Cardiovascular Exercise:

Cardiovascular exercise is essential for maintaining a healthy heart, improving endurance, and promoting overall fitness. Activities such as running, cycling, swimming or brisk walking increase the heart rate and strengthen the cardiovascular system. Regular cardiovascular exercise not only helps you maintain a healthy weight, it also increases your energy levels and reduces your risk of chronic disease. Incorporating at least 150 minutes of moderate-intensity aerobic exercise or 75 minutes of vigorous-intensity aerobic exercise into your weekly routine can make a significant contribution to your physical well-being.

## Building Strength and Muscle Tone:

Strength training is an important part of your physical well-being, especially as you age. Resistance exercises like weightlifting or bodyweight exercises help build lean muscle mass, increase bone density, and improve overall strength and stability. Strength training not only improves your physical appearance by strengthening and strengthening your muscles, it also speeds up your metabolism and promotes healthy aging. Incorporating strength training into your exercise plan two to three times a week can have significant benefits for your physical well-being.

## Flexibility and Balance:

Flexibility and balance are often overlooked aspects of physical well-being, but they are critical to maintaining mobility, preventing injury and improving overall fitness. Exercises such as yoga, Pilates, or stretching help improve flexibility, increase joint mobility, and improve balance and coordination. By focusing on these aspects, you can move more freely, improve your posture, and reduce the risk of falling or other injuries. Incorporating regular mobility and balance exercises into your daily routine can improve your physical well-being and overall quality of life.

## Pay attention to ergonomics:

The way you interact with your surroundings can have a significant impact on your physical well-being. Paying attention to ergonomics, especially in the workplace or in everyday activities, can help prevent musculoskeletal problems and promote optimal posture. Make sure your workspace is ergonomically positioned with the right desk and chair height, and take breaks throughout the day to stretch and exercise. Paying attention to your posture and body mechanics during everyday activities like lifting heavy objects or using electronic devices can help prevent overuse and injury.

## Regular check-ups:

Regular check-ups and check-ups are essential to your physical well-being. Make regular appointments with your doctor to monitor your general health, fix any problems, and get proper preventive care. This includes regular check-ups, vaccinations, screening for various medical conditions, and talking about lifestyle choices and risk factors. By putting your health first and seeking professional advice, you can identify any problems early and take proactive steps to maintain your physical well-being.

## Listen to your body's signals:

Your body is constantly sending out signals about its needs and limits. Hearing and listening to these signals is vital to your physical well-being. Pay attention to hunger and satiety signals to provide your body with the right amount of food. Take breaks and rest when you feel tired or overworked. Recognize signs of pain or discomfort and respond quickly. By creating a conscious connection with your body, you can respond to its needs more effectively and maintain your physical well-being more effectively.

## Conclusion:

Taking care of physical well-being is a multifaceted activity that requires attention to different aspects of health. Prioritizing regular exercise, nourishing the body through a healthy diet, getting adequate rest and sleep, practicing skin care and maintenance, maintaining proper posture and body language, managing stress, engaging the mind and body, strengthening and tone through cardiovascular exercise If you practice flexibility and balance, pay attention to ergonomics, schedule regular check-ups and listen to your body's signals, you can develop a strong, vibrant and resilient body. Taking care of your physical well-being is not only an investment in your attractiveness, but also a commitment to your overall health and happiness.

# Chapter No. 5

# Radiating Positive Energy

## Introduction:

In this chapter we will explore the concept of radiating positive energy to increase our attractiveness and connect with others on a deeper level. Your energy has a major impact on your interactions, relationships, and overall well-being. By cultivating and radiating positive energy, you can create a magnetic presence that draws people in and increases your sense of accomplishment.

## Developing a Positive Attitude About Yourself:

Radiating positive energy begins with developing a positive attitude and talking to yourself. Practice self-compassion, focus on your strengths, and celebrate your accomplishments. Adopt a growth mentality that sees challenges as opportunities for growth and learning. By maintaining a positive relationship with yourself, you can radiate an authentic and uplifting energy that resonates with others.

## Gratitude and Appreciation:

Expressing gratitude and appreciation is a powerful way to radiate positive energy. Take time each day to think about the things you are grateful for and express your gratitude to others. Gratitude shifts focus to the positive aspects of life and promotes a sense of fullness and contentment. When you radiate gratitude, you increase the energy around you and attract more positive experiences.

## Practicing Kindness and Compassion:

Acts of kindness and compassion have a domino effect, spreading positivity in both the giver and the receiver. Participate in other small gestures of kindness, such as a helping hand, compliments, or practice active listening. Show empathy and understanding and show compassion for yourself and others. By cultivating kindness and compassion, you create a harmonious and uplifting energy that enhances your attractiveness and strengthens your relationships.

## Cultivating Optimism:

Optimism is a powerful mindset that allows you to see the potential for positive outcomes in any situation. Cultivate optimism by turning challenges into opportunities, focusing on solutions rather than problems, and surrounding yourself with positive influences. Optimism exudes a sense of hope and possibility, makes you more approachable, and inspires positivity in others.

## Authenticity and Real Connection:

Radiating positive energy isn't about putting on a facade, it's about embracing your authentic self and truly connecting with others. Be true to yourself, express your thoughts and feelings authentically and actively listen to others without judgment. Authenticity creates an energetic resonance that fosters trust, deepens connections, and amplifies positive energy.

## Conscious Presence:

Being fully present in the moment is a powerful way to radiate positive energy. Practice mindfulness by paying attention to your surroundings, focusing on the present moment, and engaging in activities with intention and full presence.

## Creating a Positive Environment:

Your physical environment can greatly affect your energy levels and overall well-being. Create a positive and uplifting space by surrounding yourself with objects, colors and scents that evoke positive emotions. Clear the clutter in your home and work environment and bring a sense of calm and clarity. Surround yourself with positive, supportive people who cheer and inspire. Cultivating a positive environment creates a nurturing and stimulating atmosphere that supports your ability to radiate positive energy.

## Emotional Resilience and Inner Peace:

Developing emotional resilience and cultivating inner peace are essential aspects of radiating positive energy. Emotional resilience allows you to bounce back from setbacks, cope effectively with stress, and maintain a positive attitude even in difficult times. Engage in self-care activities that promote emotional well-being, such as journaling, meditation, or hobbies you enjoy. Cultivate a sense of inner peace through mindfulness practices, breathing exercises, or connecting with nature. When you embody emotional resilience and inner peace, you radiate a calming and uplifting energy that has a positive impact on those around you.

## Positive Communication:

Communication plays an important role in spreading positive energy. Focus on using positive, uplifting language when speaking to others. Practice active listening and show genuine interest in what others have to say. Pay attention to your tone of voice and body language and make sure they align with your intent to project positivity. Use words of encouragement and support to cheer and inspire those around you. Positive communication promotes a harmonious and uplifting energy in your interactions, strengthening relationships and creating a positive impact.

## Getting Rid of Negativity:

In order to release positive energy, it is important to let go of the negativity in your life. Get rid of grudges, resentments and negative attachments weighing you down. Practice forgiveness, both for others and for yourself, to free yourself from the burdens of the past. Surround yourself with positive influences and minimize exposure to negative things, be they negative news, toxic relationships, or self-limiting beliefs. By consciously choosing to let go of negativity, you create space for the positive to flourish and radiate from you.

## Encourage a sense of humor and lightness:

Humor has the unique power to uplift the spirit and create a positive atmosphere. Develop your sense of humor and learn to laugh at the ups and downs of life. Find joy in simple pleasures and master the ease in your interactions. Use humor to relieve tension, lift others' spirits, and create a positive and comfortable environment. When you exude a sense of humor and lightness, you become a source of positivity and attract others who appreciate your positive energy.

## Contributing to the Wellbeing of Others:

One of the most powerful ways to radiate positive energy is to contribute to the wellbeing of others. Participate in acts of service and kindness that encourage and support those in need. Volunteer for a cause you care about or just help someone in your community. By making a positive difference in the lives of others, you create a positive impact that extends far beyond your immediate environment.

## Continued Personal Growth:

A commitment to personal growth and self-improvement is an important aspect of radiating positive energy. Keep learning, discover new interests, and set goals that align with your values and aspirations. Treat challenges as opportunities for growth and see failures as valuable lessons. When you continuously invest in your personal development, you exude determination, enthusiasm and positive energy that inspires and motivates others.

## Positive Attitude:

A positive attitude is the basis for radiating positive energy. Train your mind to focus on the positive aspects of life and transform negative thoughts into uplifting thoughts. Practice positive affirmations and visualizations to boost your positivity. Surround yourself with positive influences, whether it's reading uplifting books, listening to inspirational podcasts, or engaging in a supportive community. A positive attitude allows you to develop an unshakeable belief in the power of positivity and transmit it to others.

## Bottom Line:

Radiating positive energy is a transformative practice that increases your attractiveness, strengthens your relationships, and contributes to your overall well-being. Cultivate a positive attitude, practice gratitude and appreciation, show kindness and compassion, embrace authenticity, be a mindful presence, cultivate a positive environment, develop emotional resilience, practice positive communication, let go of negativity, cultivate humor and lightness. Contribute to well-being. Being Others By engaging in personal development and adopting a positive attitude, you can radiate positive energy into all areas of your life. Remember that positive energy is contagious and by embodying and radiating positivity you have the power to uplift, inspire and create a more positive and harmonious world around you.

# Chapter No. 6

# Unleashing Your Inner Beauty

## Introduction:

Unleash Your Inner Beauty goes beyond your physical appearance and focuses on developing and expressing the unique qualities that make you truly beautiful from within. This chapter discusses the importance of self-discovery, self-acceptance, and self-expression in discovering one's inner beauty. By embracing and flaunting your authentic self, you can exude captivating, magnetic, and timeless beauty.

## Self-Discovery:

Unleashing your inner beauty begins with self-discovery. Take the time to explore your passions, interests, values, and beliefs. Think about what makes you happy and what makes you feel truly alive. When you discover your authentic self, you can align your life choices, actions, and relationships with who you really are. When you live in harmony with your essence, you radiate a mesmerizing and compelling natural beauty.

## Self-Acceptance:

Self-acceptance is a crucial step in unleashing your inner beauty. Accept yourself fully, including your perceived flaws and imperfections. Realize that true beauty comes from accepting and loving yourself unconditionally. Leave comparisons and societal expectations behind and celebrate your unique qualities and individuality. When you genuinely accept and love yourself, you exude confidence and inner peace, which are undeniably beautiful.

## Cultivating Inner Confidence:

Confidence is a key ingredient to unlocking inner beauty. Develop a deep self-confidence and confidence in your abilities. Focus on your strengths and achievements and let go of self-doubt and limiting beliefs. See challenges as opportunities for growth while celebrating your successes. When you radiate inner confidence, you radiate radiant energy that draws others in and inspires them to embrace their own beauty.

## Authentic Self-Expression:

Unleashing your inner beauty requires authentic self-expression. Find ways to express your creativity, be it through art, music, writing, fashion or any other form of self-expression. Embrace your unique style and personal taste and let it shine through in the way you present yourself to the world. Authentic self-expression lets your inner beauty shine through and draws others into your authentic and captivating presence.

## Embrace Emotional Intelligence:

Emotional Intelligence plays a vital role in unfolding your inner beauty. Develop your ability to understand and manage emotions, as well as to empathize with and connect deeply with others. Encourage confidence, emotional resilience, and healthy communication skills. When you embody emotional intelligence, you create meaningful connections, foster harmony in relationships, and radiate a genuine warmth and beauty that touches the hearts of those around you.

## Practicing Kindness and Empathy:

Kindness and empathy are qualities that bring out your inner beauty and have a lasting effect on others. Practice kind acts toward yourself and others, and develop genuine empathy for the experiences and feelings of those around you. Be compassionate, listen, and help if you can. When you embody kindness and empathy, you exude a beauty that is deeply felt and appreciated by others.

## Cultivating Gratitude and Positivity:

Gratitude and positivity are powerful tools for unlocking inner beauty. Cultivate a daily gratitude practice of consciously acknowledging and appreciating the blessings and abundance in your life. Focus on the positive aspects of any situation and keep a positive attitude even in difficult times. When you radiate gratitude and positivity, you radiate uplifting energy that brightens the lives of those around you.

## Maintaining Loving Relationships:

The quality of your relationships has a significant impact on your inner beauty. Maintain loving and supportive relationships with your family, friends, and loved ones. Maintain open communication, trust and mutual respect. Surround yourself with people who encourage and inspire you. When you live in warm and loving relationships, you feel seen, valued, and valued, and your inner beauty blossoms naturally.

## Inner balance and well-being:

In order to unleash inner beauty, inner balance and well-being must be cultivated. Take care of your physical, mental and emotional health. Engage in self-care activities that rejuvenate and nourish your mind, body and spirit. Rely on rest, relaxation and introspection. When you achieve inner balance and well-being, you radiate a radiant and vibrant beauty that comes from a place of self-care and self-love.

## Embrace the Connection Between Mind and Body:

To unleash your inner beauty, you must acknowledge the deep connection between body and mind. Take the time to listen to and respect your body's needs. Engage in activities that promote physical well-being, such as exercising regularly, eating a healthy diet, and getting enough rest. Cultivate mindfulness practices such as meditation or yoga to encourage mind-body connection. When you prioritize the alignment of mind and body, you radiate the beauty that emanates from a holistic place of well-being.

## Authenticity in Relationships:

Authenticity is a powerful aspect of unlocking inner beauty in relationships. Be true to yourself and express your thoughts, feelings and desires honestly and openly. Create spaces where others can be themselves. Be sensitive and let others see and recognize you. Authenticity fosters deep connections and meaningful relationships that contribute to your inner beauty and personal growth.

## Embracing Personal Passions:

Embracing and pursuing personal passions is the way to unlock inner beauty. Identify activities, hobbies, or causes that ignite and bring joy to your soul. Take the time and energy to pursue these passions on a regular basis. When you engage in activities that match your passions, you radiate a vibrant energy that exudes beauty and inspires others to follow their passions.

## Inner Strength and Resilience:

Inner strength and resilience are qualities that contribute to your inner beauty. Foster your resilience by seeing challenges as opportunities for growth and learning. Develop a mindset that sees setbacks as temporary and in the past. In difficult times, tap into your inner strength by letting it guide you through adversity. When you have inner strength and resilience, you radiate the beauty that emanates from your unwavering spirit.  ~

## Introspection and Personal Development:

Unleashing your inner beauty requires constant introspection and personal development. Take time for introspection and self-evaluation. Reflect on your values, beliefs and behaviors and identify opportunities for improvement. Participate in continuous personal development through learning, self-development and expanding your horizons. When you engage in self-reflection and personal growth, you develop a beauty that evolves and deepens over time.

## Authentic Personal Care:

Authentic Personal Care is an essential part of unfolding your inner beauty. Prioritize self-care practices that truly nourish and rejuvenate you. This can include activities such as finding quiet moments for yourself, participating in self-care rituals, setting boundaries, and practicing self-compassion. When you prioritize genuine self-care, you radiate the beauty that comes with loving and caring for yourself.

## Embracing Change and Transformation:

Embracing change and transformation is essential to unlocking the beauty within us. Life is a journey of development and evolution and acceptance of change allows you to explore new possibilities and discover hidden aspects of yourself. Use transformative experiences, whether personal, professional or in relationships, and let them shape you into a more authentic and beautiful version of yourself.

## Cultivating Inner Wisdom:

Cultivating Inner Wisdom means using your intuition and inner knowledge. Trust your instincts and listen to the wisdom within you. Connect with your intuition through exercises like meditation, journaling, or silent contemplation. When you cultivate inner wisdom, you radiate beauty that emanates from a place of deep inner knowledge and guidance.

## Accepting Imperfection:

To release inner beauty, one must accept imperfection and let go of the pursuit of perfection. Accept your flaws and realize that they are part of what makes you unique. Shift your focus from striving for perfection to accepting your authentic self. When you embrace and celebrate your imperfections, you radiate a real, relatable, and inspiring beauty.

## Summary:

Unleashing Your Inner Beauty is a multi-faceted journey that encompasses self-discovery, self-acceptance, self-expression, personal growth, and healing of the mind, body, and spirit. By embracing authenticity, cultivating inner trust, practicing kindness and empathy, prioritizing self-care, and embracing change and transformation, you can unleash authentic, compelling, and powerful beauty. Remember that your inner beauty is a reflection of your unique essence, and letting it shine inspires others to do the same.

# Chapter No. 7

# The Art of Self-Care

## Entry:

In a world where looks and first impressions count, the art of self-care is paramount. Beyond the superficial, self-care encompasses a holistic approach to self-care that aims to increase physical attractiveness and radiate an inner glow that captivates others. It's about investing time and effort to promote physical health, mental well-being and emotional balance. By immersing yourself in self-care, you begin a transformational journey that will not only make you more attractive, but also enrich your overall well-being. Let's take a closer look at the different dimensions of self-care.

## Body:

Physical health is the foundation of attractiveness, both aesthetically and vitally. Regular exercise not only helps you maintain a healthy weight, but also improves your posture, boosts your energy levels, and boosts your confidence. By combining exercise with a balanced, nutritious diet and staying hydrated, the body is nourished from the inside out, resulting in glowing skin, strong hair and overall radiance. In addition, restful sleep focuses on rejuvenating and regenerating the body, leaving you feeling refreshed and revitalized.

## Skincare:

Your skin is a canvas that deserves special attention. Introducing a skincare routine tailored to your specific skin type and concerns can do wonders for your beauty. Constantly cleansing, moisturizing and protecting your skin from the harmful effects of the sun with sunscreen is the foundation of good skin care. Regular exfoliation removes dead skin cells, unclogs pores and reveals a clear, youthful complexion. By further adapting your routine and incorporating specific anti-aging products or treatments, you can target specific issues and enhance your natural beauty. The advice of a dermatologist or skincare specialist can provide valuable information on how to achieve optimal skin health.

## Grooming:

Grooming is a key aspect of grooming that has a major impact on attractiveness. Maintaining personal hygiene through regular bathing, oral hygiene, and fresh breath is essential. Well-groomed and cared for hair, including a regular haircut and the right hair care products, will add a touch of sophistication to your look. For people with facial hair, grooming improves facial features and ensures a well-groomed appearance. Additionally, the
's attention to small details, like manicured nails and sharply sculpted eyebrows, demonstrates a meticulous approach that adds to the overall look.

## Fashion and Style:

Your clothing choices and personal style are powerful tools for self-expression and attractiveness. Dressing well means choosing clothes that flatter your figure, fit you well, and give you confidence. You can express your personality and individuality by experimenting with colours, patterns and accessories. Following fashion trends can help you keep up to date and maintain a stylish image. By choosing a wardrobe that reflects your unique style, you exude confidence and charm.

## Esprit:

Concern for your mental and emotional well-being is critical to creating attractiveness. It's important to engage in activities that bring you joy, reduce your stress, and make you feel accomplished. Whether through hobbies, creative pursuits, or mindfulness and meditation practices, these activities contribute to mental clarity and emotional balance. Seeking therapy or counseling can also be an invaluable resource in resolving underlying issues and aiding personal growth. When your mind is calm and your emotional well-being is nurtured, you exude confidence and a positive attitude that draws others magnetically to you.

## Confidence and Self-Expression:

Confidence is undeniably attractive. To build confidence, you must embrace your unique qualities and strengths, celebrate your achievements, and fully accept yourself. Engaging in activities that showcase your talents and passions, setting and achieving goals, and stepping out of your comfort zone will boost your confidence. Surround yourself with positive influences and supportive relationships that will lift your spirits and boost your confidence. By expressing yourself authentically and embracing your individuality, you radiate an irresistible charm that captivates others.

## Conclusion:

The art of self-care goes beyond superficial beauty and takes you on a profound journey of personal growth and well-being. By investing your time, effort, and dedication in self-care practices, you will unlock your true potential and increase your overall attractiveness. Prioritizing physical health, skin care, body care, and stylish clothing all contribute to your outward attractiveness. Cultivate mental and emotional well-being, develop self-confidence and self-expression.

creates an inner glow that captivates others. The transformative power of personal care lies not only in increasing attractiveness, but also in enriching the overall quality of life. Take the art of self-care as a journey of a lifetime and watch as you blossom into the most attractive and vibrant version of yourself.

# Chapter No. 8

# Developing a Growth Mindset

**Introduction:**

In today's society, attractiveness goes far beyond outward appearance. While physical beauty may initially draw a person's attention, it is often a person's mindset and inner qualities that make them truly attractive and appealing in the long run. One of the key aspects that can significantly increase a person's overall attractiveness is developing a growth mentality.

The growth mentality concept, popularized by psychologist Carol Dweck, refers to the belief that our abilities and intelligence can be developed through dedication, hard work, and a willingness to learn. People with a growth mentality see challenges as opportunities for growth and failures as valuable learning experiences. You are open to feedback, resistant to mistakes and strive to constantly improve.

By developing a growth mindset you can change your life and become a more attractive and attractive person. This way of thinking affects not only your self-image, but also the way you interact with others and how you approach personal and professional development. In this article, we explore the different ways to develop a growth mentality and use its power to become more attractive to others.

## Facing Challenges and New Experiences:

 Focus on growth encourages you to step out of your comfort zone and see challenges as opportunities for personal growth. By welcoming new experiences, whether it's learning a new skill, taking on a challenging project, or participating in unfamiliar social situations, you show a willingness to continue developing and expanding your skills. This openness to challenges not only helps you develop new skills, but also demonstrates your confidence and adaptability, which makes you more attractive and interesting to others.

## Cultivating a Positive Attitude and Resilience:

 The Growth Mindset emphasizes the power of positivity and resilience in the face of obstacles. Rather than doubting or giving up in the face of setbacks, people with a growth mindset stay positive and see challenges as opportunities for personal growth. This optimism and resilience are very attractive traits because they demonstrate your ability to face adversity with grace and recover from setbacks, and inspire others around you to adopt a similar mindset.

## Lifelong Learning:

A growth mentality fosters a deep commitment to continuous learning and improvement. By adopting a mindset that values lifelong learning, you demonstrate intellectual curiosity, humility, and a willingness to expand your knowledge and skills. Commitment to continuing education, pursuing personal hobbies and interests, and seeking development opportunities not only increases your attractiveness but also makes you a more committed and well-rounded individual.

## Focus on Effort and Perseverance:

In a growth mindset, effort and perseverance are considered essential success factors. By valuing and prioritizing hard work, people with a growth mentality show commitment and determination. This focus on effort rather than solely relying on innate talent or ability demonstrates your work ethic and dedication, which are very attractive traits in personal and professional contexts.

## Accept feedback and surround yourself with positive influences:

Growth mentality is based on feedback and ideas from others. Get opinions and actively listen to others. You are open to development and improvement. Additionally, being surrounded by positive influences like mentors, supportive friends, and like-minded peers can boost your growth mindset, giving you the encouragement and inspiration to grow and grow as you grow.

## Conclusion:

Developing a growth mentality is a powerful tool that can significantly increase your attractiveness both in your personal relationships and in your professional projects. By accepting challenges, maintaining a positive attitude, encouraging a willingness to learn, emphasizing effort and perseverance, and seeking positive feedback and positive influences, you can become more engaging and attractive. Remember that attractiveness goes beyond looks. Developing a growth mindset can make you compelling and showcase your potential for growth, resilience, and continuous self-improvement. .

# Chapter No. 9

# Letting Go of Comparison and Society's Standards

**Voice:**

In today's society, the pressure to conform to certain beauty standards and ideals can be overwhelming. From flawless Photoshop photos in magazines to carefully curated social media profiles, we are constantly bombarded with images and messages telling us how we should look and what is considered attractive. Not surprisingly, many people struggle with their self-esteem and body image when trying to live up to these unrealistic expectations.

The real appeal, however, goes far beyond narrow societal definitions. It's about accepting and loving yourself for who you are, both inside and out. It's about recognizing your unique qualities and freeing yourself from the need to compare yourself to others. By changing our perspective and focusing on self-acceptance and self-development, we can become more attractive in ways that go beyond just our looks.

In this article we will examine the importance of rejecting social comparisons and norms in order to increase our attractiveness. We discuss practical strategies for cultivating self-love, accepting self-esteem, and building self-confidence. When we understand that beauty takes many forms and cannot be confined to societal expectations, we can embark on a journey of self-discovery and transformation that radiates true attractiveness from within. So let's take a look at the process of increasing attractiveness by rejecting social comparisons and norms.

## Recognizing the Harmful Effects of Comparison:

Comparison is a natural human tendency that often arises from a desire for recognition and acceptance. However, when it comes to our self-esteem and attractiveness, constant comparison can have negative effects. This leads to feelings of inadequacy, insecurity, and a distorted self-image. Comparison to others, especially based on social norms, creates unrealistic expectations and perpetuates a cycle of dissatisfaction. It's important to recognize the harm that comparison can do and to understand that our worth does not depend on how we compare ourselves to others.

## Use Your Unique Qualities:

Everyone has a unique combination of qualities, talents and attributes that make them valuable in themselves. When you accept your uniqueness, you appreciate and celebrate what makes you different. Take the time to discover your passions, strengths and interests. By focusing on your individuality, you can increase your attractiveness while exuding confidence and authenticity. Remember that true beauty is embracing and expressing your true self and not trying to fit into society's patterns.

## Focus on Inner Beauty:

While outward appearances often draw the most attention, it's important to realize that true attractiveness goes beyond outward appearances. Inner beauty, made up of qualities like kindness, compassion, empathy, and self-confidence, has a significant impact on how we see ourselves and others. When we prioritize cultivating these qualities, we radiate a magnetic energy that draws people to us. By appreciating and nurturing our inner beauty, we can build meaningful relationships with others based on genuine qualities and not superficial judgments.

## Practicing Self-Love and Caring:

Self-love and self-care are essential practices for increasing overall attractiveness and well-being. Cultivating self-love involves unconditional self-acceptance, accepting our strengths and weaknesses, and treating ourselves with kindness and compassion. Equally important is engaging in self-care activities that promote physical, emotional, and spiritual well-being. This can include activities such as regular exercise, eating a balanced diet, getting enough rest, pursuing hobbies, and seeking support from loved ones Confidence that others find attractive.

## Surrounding Yourself with Positive Influences:

The people and media we surround ourselves with have a major impact on our perception of ourselves and our attractiveness. Surrounding ourselves with uplifting people who value and celebrate our uniqueness can create a positive environment conducive to personal growth. Additionally, exploring different representations of beauty in media and social media can help challenge narrow standards of beauty. It is also important not to expose yourself to negative influences that perpetuate unrealistic ideals. By leading a positive and supportive Circle, we create an environment that fosters our self-esteem and encourages us to embrace our authentic selves.

## Setting Realistic Goals and Celebrating Progress:

Setting realistic goals that align with our values and aspirations is a step toward personal development. Remember that progress is more valuable than perfection. By breaking bigger goals down into smaller, achievable steps, we can track our progress and celebrate each step along the way. This approach promotes a sense of accomplishment and boosts self-confidence, making us more attractive to others and, most importantly, to ourselves. When we embark on a journey of self-improvement and appreciating our progress, we radiate an inner confidence that draws others to us.

## Conclusion:

Letting go of comparisons and social norms is a transformative process that requires self-reflection, self-acceptance, and a change in mindset. By acknowledging the harmful effects of comparison, embracing our unique qualities, focusing on our inner beauty, practicing self-love and self-care, surrounding ourselves with positive influences, and setting realistic goals, we can free ourselves from the constraints of societal expectations. In this way we unfold our true attractiveness, which results from self-acceptance, authenticity and self-development. Appreciate your uniqueness, celebrate your journey and watch your charm radiate from within, captivating those around you.

# Chapter No. 10

# Discovering Your Personal Style

## Introducing:

Discovering and embracing your own style is a transformative journey that goes beyond simple fashion choices. It is a process of self-expression, self-discovery and self-confidence. Your personal style reflects your interior, your uniqueness and your individuality. When you align your outward appearance with your authentic self, you not only increase your attractiveness, but also promote a sense of self-determination and personal fulfillment. In this article, we dive into the process of discovering your style and how it can contribute to your overall attractiveness and well-being.

## Understanding the Importance of Personal Style:

Personal style is not just about following trends or conforming to societal expectations. It's about embracing your true self and expressing your identity through your looks. Your personal style serves as a visual representation of your personality, values, and tastes. When you dress to fit you, you're sending a powerful message to the world that you're confident, authentic, and good about yourself. Recognizing the importance of personal style allows
to approach the process consciously and use it as a path to independence.

## Thinking About Your Personality and Lifestyle:

To discover your personal style, take the time for self-reflection and self-exploration. Consider your personality traits, interests, passions, and values. Think about how you want to present yourself to the world and what message you want to convey with your style. Consider your lifestyle, including daily activities, work environment, and community involvement. By thinking about these aspects, you can tailor the style to your unique characteristics and create a coherent and authentic
image.

## Explore different fashion styles and inspiration:

Fashion is an ever-changing landscape with a variety of styles and aesthetics. Take the opportunity to explore different fashion styles and find inspiration that speaks to you. Look for style icons, fashion influencers and celebrities whose style you admire. Browse fashion magazines, blogs and social media platforms for ideas. Pay attention to the elements, colors, patterns and silhouettes that you like the most. Remember, personal style isn't about copying someone else's look, it's about incorporating elements that inspire you into your own unique expression.

## Build a versatile and cohesive wardrobe:

Building a versatile wardrobe is key to effectively expressing your style. First, evaluate your existing wardrobe and select items that no longer fit your desired style. Focus on getting the necessary pieces that can be combined to create a variety of outfits. Invest in quality basics like skinny jeans, slim-fit blazers, versatile suits and classic shirts. When choosing clothes, consider your body shape, color palette, and personal preferences. Try to find a balance between timeless classics and trendier elements to keep your wardrobe eclectic and current.

## Pay Attention to Appearance and Presentation:

Personal style isn't just about clothes; This includes grooming and self-introduction. Take care of your physical appearance by following a skin care routine that suits your skin type and improves your complexion. Experiment with different hairstyles, hair colors, and makeup to find ones that suit your facial features and style. Pay attention to grooming details such as well-trimmed nails, clean and waxed shoes, and proper hygiene practices.
Remember that your personal style is an overall expression of yourself and how you present yourself to the world can have a huge impact on your overall attractiveness.

## Cultivating Trust and Authenticity:

The essence of personal style is the trust and authenticity with which you carry yourself. Accept your choices and wear your outfits with pride and conviction. Let your personal style be a tool for self-expression and self-acceptance. When you feel confident and authentic in what you wear, it radiates through your body language, behavior, and interactions with others. Develop a sense of security, celebrate your individuality and let your style become part of your identity.

## Summary:

Discovering and embracing your own style is a profound journey that will enable you to express your true personality and increase your attractiveness. This includes understanding the importance of personal style as a means of expression and empowerment. By thinking about your personality, exploring different fashion styles, building a versatile wardrobe, paying attention to appearance and self-expression, and cultivating self-confidence and authenticity, you can create a unique style team. Embark on this journey of self-discovery and let your personal style become a powerful tool to reveal your inner beauty and captivate those around you. Remember that the most attractive version of you is the one that reflects your true essence.

# Chapter No. 11

# Dressing to Enhance Your Features

Dressing to highlight your facial features is a great way to increase your attractiveness and bring out your best features. By choosing the right clothing styles, colors and cuts, you can create a flattering and confident look that brings out your natural beauty.

Here are some tips for clothing that flatters your assets:

## Know Your Body Type:

In order to choose clothes that flatter your figure, it is important to know your body type. Whether you have an hourglass, pear, apple or athletic figure, there are certain styles that can highlight your best features. Discover different body types and find out which clothing silhouettes suit you best.

## Highlight Your Strengths:

 Identify the parts of your body that you love and want to pay attention to. If you have shapely legs, consider wearing skirts or dresses that show them off. If you have a small waist, choose belted or fitted tops to accentuate it. By highlighting your best qualities, you can create a more appealing overall look.

## Color Coordination:

Choosing the right colors can significantly transform your appearance. Find out which colors match your skin tone, hair color and eye color. For example, if you have a warm complexion, earth tones like browns, oranges, and warm greens can be flattering. If you have cool undertones, blue, purple, and jewel tones can suit you well. Experiment with different color palettes to find what makes you vibrant and radiant.

## Dress appropriately for the occasion:

Be aware of the context in which you are dressing. A dress appropriate to the occasion can make you more attractive and beautiful. Whether it's a formal event, a casual outing, or a work atmosphere, choose clothing that conforms to the dress code while still reflecting your personal style.

## Find the right size:

Clothing that doesn't fit you can instantly ruin your overall image. Make sure your clothes fit you well and flatter your figure. Avoid clothing that is too tight or too loose, as either extreme can be unfavorable. The way your clothes fit your body can have a significant impact on how you look and feel.

## Pay attention to the details:

Small details in your outfit can make a big difference to your overall impression. Consider accessories like jewelry, belts, scarves, and handbags to add interest and style to your look. But remember, moderation is key. Don't overload your outfit with too many accessories; Instead, pick a word element or two to improve your overall look.

## Dress Confidently:

Ultimately, the most attractive thing you can wear is confidence. When you're comfortable with what you're wearing, it shows in your demeanor and body language. Wear clothes that make you feel comfortable, stylish, and true to yourself. Confidence is contagious and makes you more attractive to others.

## Highlight your most beautiful features:

Your choice of clothing can also draw attention to your facial features. If you have beautiful eyes, you should wear blouses or accessories that emphasize their color. For example, a complementary shade of blue in your outfit can make blue eyes stand out. If you have high cheekbones, try hairstyles that keep the hair out of your face or wear low-cut tops to emphasize the feature.

## Consider proportions:

 Proportions play a crucial role in how clothes look on the body. If you have a long torso, high-waist pants can help create the illusion of longer legs. If you have a shorter torso, choose pants with a low waist to balance the proportions. Be aware of where the clothes sit on your body and experiment with different cuts and lengths to find what works best for you.

## Using Templates Strategically:

Templates can be used to emphasize or distract from specific areas of the body. Eye-catching patterns and prints usually draw attention. So if you want to highlight a specific area, choose patterned clothing for that specific part. Conversely, if you want to minimize an area, choose solid colors or smaller, more subtle patterns in that area.

## Pay attention to your choice of fabric:

The fabric of your clothes can affect their fit and your overall comfort. Lighter fabrics like silk or chiffon can create a softer, more sophisticated look, while textured fabrics like tweed or denim can add definition and shape. Choose fabrics that suit your body type and the desired outcome with your outfit.

## Experiment with layering:

Layering can add depth and dimension to an outfit while allowing you to mix and match different pieces. By strategically arranging your clothes, you can create interesting combinations that enhance your overall look. For example, wearing a well-tailored blazer over a blouse can instantly elevate your look and give it a more sophisticated appeal.

## Pay attention to the footwear:

The choice of your footwear can have a big impact on your overall appearance. Wearing heels can lengthen your legs and improve your posture, making you look taller and more confident. However, if you don't feel comfortable in high heels, there are many options for stylish flats that can elevate your outfit. Choose shoes that match your outfit and provide the right level of comfort for the occasion.

## Cultivate Good Grooming Habits:

No matter how well-dressed you are, cultivating good grooming habits is important to increasing your overall attractiveness. Keep your hair in good condition, keep your nails neat and tidy, and take care of your skin.

Remember that the purpose of clothing that flatters your features is to create a harmonious and confident image that reflects your personal style. It's about feeling good about yourself and accepting your own unique qualities. Use these tips as a guide, but always trust your instincts and preferences when it comes to choosing clothes that make you feel attractive and powerful.

# Chapter No. 12

# Grooming for Self-Expression

Personal hygiene is not just about personal hygiene; It is also an opportunity to express yourself and increase your attractiveness. The way you get married can express your style, personality and confidence.

Here are some ways grooming can express your personality and increase your attractiveness:

## Hair Care:

Your hairstyle can have a significant impact on your overall appearance. Experiment with different hairstyles, colors, and styles that suit your face shape and personal style. Whether you prefer a sleek, elegant look or a more relaxed, messy look, healthy, well-groomed hair can instantly boost your attractiveness. Remember to use the right hair products and tools to keep your hair looking its best.

## Skin Care:

Taking care of your skin not only makes you look healthy, it also gives you confidence. Establish a skincare routine that suits your skin type and concerns, including cleansing, moisturizing, and using sunscreen. Consider using other products like serums or masks to address your skin's specific needs. When your skin is clean, radiant and nourished, it enhances your overall attractiveness and makes you look fresh and youthful.

## Beard Grooming:

Whether you prefer a clean-shaven look or a sporty stubble look, beard or mustache grooming can add a touch of personality to your look. Make sure your stubble is properly trimmed, shaped and groomed to keep it looking clean and shiny. Experiment with different styles and lengths depending on your face shape and personal style.

## Nail care:

Well-groomed nails can contribute to a shiny and attractive overall appearance. Keep your nails clean, trimmed and shaped. If you prefer to wear nail polish, choose colors that complement your skin tone and clothing choices. Moisturize your hands and cuticles regularly to keep them healthy and prevent dryness.

## Personal hygiene:

pay attention to the small details of personal hygiene, e.g. For example, keeping your breath clean and fresh, using deodorant or antiperspirant, and making sure your clothes are clean and well-ironed. These seemingly insignificant aspects can have a huge impact on your overall attractiveness and make a positive impression on others.

## Perfume:

Wearing a pleasant perfume can increase your charm and leave a lasting impression. Find a fragrance that suits your personality and complements your body chemistry. Experiment with different scents like floral, woody, or citrusy scents to find what works best for you. Remember to apply perfume sparingly, concentrating on pulse points like the wrists and neck.

## Oral Hygiene:

A healthy and confident smile can instantly increase your attractiveness. Maintain good oral hygiene by brushing your teeth at least twice a day, flossing regularly, and using mouthwash. Schedule regular dental check-ups to make sure your teeth and gums are in good shape.

## Grooming:

Pay attention to general grooming to promote a healthy and attractive appearance. This includes regular baths or showers, using moisturizers to keep the skin hydrated, and using appropriate personal care products. Remember to wear clean, well-fitting clothing that flatters your figure and personal style.

Remember in order to prepare for self-expression, you must accept your individuality and present yourself in a way that makes you confident and attractive. Experiment with different techniques, products, and styles to see what works for you. Taking the time to take care of yourself and expressing your personal style through grooming can have a positive impact on your self-esteem and how others see you.

## Makeup for Self-Expression:

Makeup can be a powerful tool for self-expression and natural facial features. Experiment with different looks that reflect your personality and style. Whether you prefer a natural, minimal look or like to experiment with bold, colorful makeup, you'll find techniques that will bring out your best features. Concentrate on emphasizing the eyes, lips or cheekbones and create a look with make-up that gives you confidence and expresses your individuality.

## Eyebrow care:

Well-groomed eyebrows can frame your face and improve your overall appearance. Determine the shape of your brows that suits your face shape, and consider techniques like tweezing, twirling, or waxing to maintain their shape and remove unwanted hair. Fill in brows with products like brow pencils or powder to define and fill in sparse areas.

## Grooming:

Grooming goes beyond personal hygiene and can be a way of expressing yourself. Decide how you style or want to style your hair based on your preferences and what gives you confidence. Whether you want to leave your hair natural or prefer to have it removed or trimmed, make sure you do it safely and in a manner that suits your personal style and comfort.

## Personal Perfume:

Your personal perfume can be a powerful way to express yourself and make a lasting impression. Find a distinctive scent or experiment with different scents that suit your personality and evoke the vibe you want to convey. Consider researching niche perfumes or artisanal perfumes to find unique scents that reflect your individuality and set you apart.

## Experiment with hairstyles:

Your hairstyle is a great way to express yourself and can transform your overall appearance. Try different hairstyles from updos to braids to loose waves that suit your personal style and the image you want to present. Consider consulting a hairstylist for recommendations based on your face shape, hair texture, and lifestyle. Don't be afraid to step out of your comfort zone and try new hairstyles that reflect your personality and make
attractive.

## Embracing Individuality:

Expressing yourself through caring is about capitalizing on your unique qualities and celebrating what sets you apart. Don't try to conform to societal norms or trends that don't match your personal style. Instead, focus on your authentic and confident expression. Use body care to bring out your individuality and personal taste and talents.

## Practice Self-Care:

In addition to your grooming routine, prioritize self-care to increase your overall attractiveness. Get enough sleep, eat a balanced diet, exercise regularly, and manage stress effectively. Taking care of your overall wellbeing will shine through your appearance and add to your attractiveness. Remember to feed yourself emotionally, engage in activities you enjoy, and keep a positive attitude.

The preparation for self-expression is a journey of self-discovery and self-care. It's about finding grooming practices and styles that fit your personality and make you feel safe and attractive. Experiment, be open to new things, and trust your gut when it comes to expressing yourself through caring. Feeling good about how you present yourself can have a positive impact on your self-esteem and how you are perceived by others.

# Chapter No. 13

# Communicating with Impact and Authenticity

Impressive and authentic communication is an effective way to increase your attractiveness. Your words, your tone of voice, your body language and your overall appearance can make a huge difference in how others perceive you. Here are some key ways to improve your communication skills and make a lasting impression:

## Active Listening:

 One of the most important aspects of effective communication is active listening. Show genuine interest in what others have to say, make eye contact, and join the conversation. Avoid interruptions and really listen to understand instead of waiting your turn to speak. Active listening shows respect, empathy, and caring, making you a more engaged conversationalist.

## Verbal communication:

When communicating verbally, pay attention to the choice of words, tone of voice and message. Pay attention to your language with clear and concise sentences. Use positive and encouraging words to create a friendly and approachable atmosphere. Practice speaking confidently and avoid mumbling or speaking too softly. A clear and confident voice can captivate others and make you more attractive in social interactions.

## Nonverbal Communication:

Nonverbal cues play an important role in communication. Pay attention to your body language, posture and gestures. Stand or sit upright in an open, relaxed posture that expresses confidence and readiness. Use an appropriate facial expression that matches the message you are conveying. Maintain eye contact, but remember to give others space and not stare too hard. Nonverbal cues that match your words create a sense of authenticity and make you more attractive to others.

## Emotional Intelligence:

Develop your emotional intelligence to understand and effectively manage your own emotions and those of others. Be aware of others' emotions and respond with empathy. Show compassion and understanding and avoid judgment and defense. Emotional intelligence allows you to connect with others on a deeper level, nurture meaningful relationships, and make you more attractive as a person.

## Authenticity:

Stay true to yourself and communicate authentically. People are attracted to people who are sincere and honest in their dealings. Don't try to be someone you're not or pretend you have qualities you don't have. Accept your unique personality, share your thoughts and opinions respectfully, and feel comfortable expressing your true self. Authenticity creates a sense of trust and attraction because it allows others to connect with the real you.

Empathy and Understanding: Practice empathy and try to understand different points of view. Show genuine concern for others' feelings and experiences and try to see the world from their perspective. Ask questions to deepen your understanding and actively empathize with their feelings. By showing empathy and understanding, you will become a compassionate and engaging communicator who builds strong bonds with others.

## Positive Body Language:

Developing positive body language can make you more attractive to others. Smile sincerely and often, as this signals openness and warmth. Use open and friendly gestures, such as nodding or leaning in slightly, when others are talking. Avoid crossing your arms or adopting defensive postures as this impedes communication. Positive body language helps create a positive and engaging atmosphere and makes you more attractive to those around you.

## Confidence:

 Confidence is an attractive quality that can greatly influence communication. Believe in yourself and your abilities, and let that confidence shine through your interactions. Speak confidently, maintain eye contact, and stand up. However, make sure that your confidence is balanced with humility and openness towards others. ideas. True trust attracts people and makes you more attractive as a communicator.

## Storytelling:

Master the art of storytelling to engage and engage your audience. Stories have the unique ability to convey emotion, connect people and leave a lasting impression. Share anecdotes or personal experiences relevant to the conversation. Use descriptive language and vivid imagery to paint a picture and evoke emotion. Storytelling allows you to communicate with depth and authenticity, which makes you more attractive as a communicator.

## Clarity and Concise:

Try to be clear and concise in communication. Before you speak, organize your thoughts and make sure your message is coherent and easy to understand. Avoid technical jargon or overly complex language that may mislead or alienate others. Present your ideas in a logical and structured way that is easy for others to understand. Clear and concise communication is a sign of respect for others. Time and attention, which makes you more attractive as a communicator.

## Empowering Others:

Make a conscious effort to empower and empower those around you through your communications. Give sincere compliments and express your appreciation for others. contribute and give constructive feedback in a positive and encouraging way. Be generous in praising, acknowledging, and expressing gratitude for the efforts of others. When you empower and encourage others, you create a positive and inclusive environment that makes you more attractive as a communicator.

## Adaptability:

Adapt your communication style to different situations and people. Recognize that everyone has different communication preferences and adjust your approach accordingly. Listen for verbal and non-verbal cues to gauge the level of formality or informality required. Adaptability shows that you are observant and flexible, which makes you more attractive as a communicator able to connect with a variety of people.

## Sensitivity to Trust:

While trust is important in communication, it is equally important to embrace vulnerability. Share your thoughts, experiences and feelings authentically, even if it makes you feel vulnerable. By showing vulnerability, you create a sense of trust and authenticity, and invite others to open up and connect with you on a deeper level. The balance between trust and vulnerability makes you more attractive as a communicator you can relate to and trust.

## Mindful Communication:

 Practice mindful communication by being fully present and aware of the moment. Avoid distractions and give your full attention to the person you are interacting with. Listen actively, think about your answers before you speak, and be thoughtful rather than impulsive. Conscious communication fosters meaningful connections, shows respect, and makes you more attractive as a communicator who appreciates and appreciates others.

## Get feedback and continuous improvement:

Actively get feedback on your communication skills to identify opportunities for improvement. Ask friends, colleagues, or trusted mentors for constructive criticism and use it as an opportunity to grow. Be open to feedback and strive to continuously improve your communication skills. A desire to learn and grow as a communicative person makes you more attractive because it shows your commitment to personal and interpersonal development.

Remember that effective communication is a lifelong journey of learning and improvement. By developing your communication skills and focusing on impact and authenticity, you can make a positive and lasting impression on others. Cultivate genuine connections, inspire others with your words, and strive to communicate powerfully and authentically in all areas of your life.

# Chapter No. 14

# The Art of Active Listening

The art of active listening is a powerful tool that can greatly increase your attractiveness as a communicator and create meaningful connections with others. Active listening goes beyond just listening to what someone is saying. it requires presence, commitment and total empathy.

Here are some important things to keep in mind as you master the art of active listening:

## Give Your Undivided Attention:

When engaged in a conversation, give your full attention to the other party. Minimize distractions by putting down the phone, turning off the TV, or finding a quiet place to focus on the conversation. Through your actions and body language, show that you are fully present and willing to listen.

## Maintain Eye Contact:

Eye contact is an essential aspect of active listening. Show respect, interest and attention. Maintain good eye contact with the speaker, but be careful not to stare too hard as this could be awkward. By looking directly at the speaker, you show that you care about what they are saying and that you value what they have to say.

## Use Nonverbal Cues:

Nonverbal cues like nodding, smiling, and leaning forward slightly can signal your commitment and understanding. These signals show that you are actively following the conversation and engaging with the speaker's message. Mirroring the speaker's body language to some extent can also create a sense of understanding and put them at ease.

## Avoid Interruptions:

An interruption can be perceived as disrespectful and disrupt the speaker's train of thought. Allow the speaker to fully express their ideas before offering your contribution. Be patient and wait for natural pauses or pauses in the conversation to step in or ask clarifying questions. By giving the speaker a chance to share their thoughts without being disturbed, you create an atmosphere of respect and caring.

## Practice Empathy:

Empathy is a fundamental part of active listening. Put yourself in the speaker's shoes and try to understand their point of view, their emotions and their experiences. Listen with an open mind and disregard your judgment or prejudices. Show empathy through your facial expressions, tone of voice, and reactions, and show them that you genuinely care about their feelings and perspective.

## Reflection and Paraphrase:

To show that you are actively listening and understanding, occasionally think about what the speaker said. Paraphrase their words or summarize their main points to make sure you get the intended message. This not only confirms your understanding, but shows that you are involved in conversations and committed to effective communication.

## Ask Open-Ended Questions:

Encourage deeper dialogue and exploration by asking open-ended questions. These questions encourage the speaker to go into more depth and detail, leading to a more intense conversation. Open-ended questions show your genuine interest in the speaker's thoughts and encourage them to share more, creating space for meaningful connection and understanding.

## Avoid Distractions and Prejudices:

Be aware of your own biases, assumptions, and distractions that may prevent you from actively listening. Approach the conversation with an open mind, free from preconceived notions or personal intentions. Really focus on what the speaker is saying instead of formulating or thinking ahead to your response. By putting aside distractions and prejudice, you can listen more actively.

## Show Appreciation and Appreciation:

Show your appreciation for the respondent's willingness to share their thoughts and feelings. Offer them validation and recognition of their ideas, even if you don't necessarily agree with everything they say. Show respect for their unique perspective and let them know their contribution is valuable. This creates a positive, affirmative environment that fosters deeper connections and encourages open communication.

## Practice Patience:

Active listening requires patience, as the speaker may need time to fully express their thoughts and feelings. Avoid rushing the conversation or trying to steer it in a different direction. Give the speaker the space and time they need to express themselves fully, allowing for a more meaningful and inclusive exchange of ideas.

## Suspension of Judgment:

Active listening requires not passing judgment and avoiding the impulse to immediately form an opinion or assumption. Instead, approach the conversation with an open mind and genuine curiosity to understand the speaker's point of view. Be aware of any prejudice or prejudice that might prevent you from listening objectively. By putting judgment aside, you create a safe, non-threatening space for open dialogue and encourage the speaker to speak freely.

## Mirror Practice:

Mirroring is a technique for mirroring the speaker's emotions and body language. By mirroring the speaker, you create a sense of empathy and connection. Pay attention to their tone of voice, facial expressions, and gestures, and mimic their behaviors subtly. However, it is important to be authentic when mirroring and not to over-mimic the speaker. Reflexivity builds a relationship and helps the speaker feel understood and valued.

## Be patient with silence:

Use moments of silence when speaking. Silence can be uncomfortable for some, but it can also be an occasion for reflection and deeper reflection. Allow the speaker to gather their thoughts and process their feelings. Avoid filling in silences with your own words or rushing to fill in gaps in the conversation. Sometimes the deepest insights and revelations come in moments of stillness.

## Practicing Mindfulness:

Engage in mindful listening by being fully present in the moment and focusing your attention on the speaker. Be aware of your thoughts, emotions, and body sensations and don't let the conversation distract you. Mindfulness helps you connect to the speaker's words and nonverbal cues, allowing you to respond in a more thoughtful and empathetic manner. Cultivating mindfulness improves your active listening and deepens your connection with other people.

## Follow up and follow up:

Active listening doesn't stop with the conversation itself. Show your commitment to the speaker's thoughts and feelings by following and implementing the actions or commitments discussed in the interview. Pay attention to the key points, tasks, or requests of the speaker and make sure you address them appropriately. Not only does this strengthen your active listening skills, but it also builds your trustworthiness and credibility as a
communicator.

## Practice self-reflection:

 Regularly reflect on your listening habits and identify opportunities for improvement. Be aware of habits or behaviors that can get in the way of effective listening, such as B. Interrupting, daydreaming, or concentrating on your response rather than the speaker's words. Actively work to overcome these obstacles and develop better listening habits. Engage in self-reflection to cultivate your self-awareness and continuously improve your active listening skills.

## Ask for feedback:

Ask others for feedback on your listening skills. Reach out to a trusted friend, colleague, or mentor and ask them to give you an honest assessment of your active listening skills. Their insights can provide valuable insights and help identify blind spots or areas where further improvements can be made. Actively seeking feedback shows your commitment to growth and development as a communicator.

## Practice empathy beyond words:

While active listening is about understands the speaker's words, it is also about noticing their feelings and hidden messages. Pay attention to the speaker's tone of voice, body language, and general demeanor to gauge their emotional state. Respond with empathy by acknowledging and validating their feelings. Show that you genuinely care about their well-being and invest in their thoughts and feelings.

## Be aware of cultural differences:

 Remember that active listening can vary from culture to culture. Different cultures can have different communication styles, expectations and norms. Be sensitive to these differences and adjust your active listening approach accordingly. Avoid making assumptions based on your cultural background and instead be open to learning about and understanding the speaker's cultural nuances.

## Take care of yourself:

Active listening can be mentally and emotionally draining, especially during intense or intense conversations. Prioritize self-care to ensure you're in a good mood and have the energy to actively listen. Participate in activities that help you relax, rejuvenate and maintain your well-being. When you take care of yourself, you can be fully present and attentive while actively listening to others.

By developing your active listening skills, you can have a profound impact on your interactions with others. Active listening increases your attractiveness as a communicator, deepens your relationships, and fosters a sense of connection and understanding. Keep practicing and perfecting the art of active listening, and you'll see how it positively impacts your personal and professional interactions.

# Chapter No. 15

# Building Meaningful Connections

Making meaningful connections is a key aspect of increasing your fascination with others. Meaningful connections go beyond superficial interactions and create a sense of genuine mutual understanding, trust and respect. Here are some ways to expand your reach to make meaningful connections:

**Authenticity:**

Be authentic and true to yourself when interacting with others. Use your strengths, weaknesses and unique traits. Avoid impersonating someone you are not. When you are authentic, you create an atmosphere of trust and openness so that others feel comfortable being authentic.

## Active Listening:

Making meaningful connections starts with being an active listener. Really participate in conversations by showing genuine interest in what others have to say. Practice the art of active listening by paying full attention, maintaining eye contact, and responding thoughtfully. By actively listening, you signal that you value the thoughts and experiences of others, thereby fostering deeper connections.

## Empathy and Compassion:

Cultivate empathy and compassion in your interactions. Try to understand the perspectives, feelings, and experiences of others. Put yourself in their shoes and acknowledge their feelings. Show empathy by offering support, encouragement, and a non-judgmental ear. Compassion fosters feelings of connectedness and helps build meaningful relationships based on mutual understanding and caring.

## Shared Interests and Passions:

Find common interests or passions with others to create shared experiences and deeper connections. Discover activities or topics that spark your passion and look for people who share those interests. Participate in discussions, participate in group activities, or join communities focused on these shared passions. Shared experiences strengthen the bond between individuals and form the basis for the development of meaningful connections.

## Sensitivity and Trust:

Making meaningful connections often requires being sensitive and building trust. Share your thoughts, feelings and experiences honestly with others and allow them to see your true self. Be open to sensitivity and encourage others to do the same. By creating a safe space for sensitivity, you build trust and deepen your connection with those around you.

## Mutual Support and Encouragement:

Support and encourage one another in your interactions. Celebrate the accomplishments and achievements of others and lend a helping hand during difficult times. Show genuine interest in their goals and desires and offer help or advice if needed. By being a source of support, you nurture a sense of camaraderie and build valuable relationships based on mutual respect and caring.

## Shared Experiences and Memories:

Participate in activities and create memories with others. This may include participating in group tours, traveling, attending events, or just eating together. Shared experiences create lasting bonds and provide opportunities to share stories and laugh. These shared memories become the basis of a shared story and foster a deeper sense of connection.

## Openness and Acceptance:

Approach interactions with an open mind and a willingness to learn from others. Embrace diversity and different perspectives and recognize that everyone has a unique background and range of experiences. Accept other opinions, even if they differ from yours. This openness and acceptance creates an inclusive environment in which valuable relationships can flourish.

## Cultivate reciprocity:

Making meaningful connections is a two-way street. Maintain reciprocity in your relationships by actively contributing to the connection. Be observant, supportive, and participate in the lives of others. Take a genuine interest in their well-being and be available when they need someone they can rely on. By nurturing reciprocity, you create a balanced and mutually beneficial connection.

## Nurture Long-Term Relationships:

Building meaningful relationships takes constant effort and nurturing. Invest time and energy in nurturing relationships by stopping by regularly, setting up meetings, or having meaningful conversations. Show your commitment to the relationship by being dependable, trustworthy, and trustworthy. Long-term relationships provide a sense of stability, understanding, and continuity, deepening the connection over time.

## Practicing sensitivity:

In order to make valuable connections, it is important to be sensitive and to be seen as authentic. Share your hopes, fears, dreams, successes and failures with others. In this way, openness creates an atmosphere of trust and encourages others to reciprocate, deepen connections, and develop a sense of emotional closeness.

## Show Your Appreciation and Gratitude:

When you express your appreciation and gratitude to others, you strengthen the bond between people. Recognize and thank people for their contributions, support, or acts of kindness. This simple act of gratitude not only shows that you value and appreciate their efforts, but also fosters a positive and uplifting atmosphere in your relationships.

## Practicing active empathy:

Empathy is about putting yourself in another person's shoes and understanding their feelings and experiences. Actively practice empathy by actively listening, observing nonverbal cues, and trying to understand the emotions behind a person's words. Show compassion and support, and offer words of comfort or encouragement when needed. This empathetic approach helps build deeper connections and encourages understanding and camaraderie.

## Develop a sense of belonging:

Create an inclusive and friendly environment where people feel they belong. Participate in your conversations, activities and decisions. Make sure every voice is heard and respected. By developing a sense of belonging, you create a space where people feel valued, accepted, and connected.

## Engage in active collaboration:

Collaboration and teamwork can strengthen bonds and create meaningful connections. Look for opportunities to collaborate with others on common projects, initiatives, or goals. When people work together to achieve a common goal, there is a sense of camaraderie, trust, and shared results.

## Don't forget non-verbal communication:

Non-verbal communication such as body language, facial expressions and gestures play an important role in forming meaningful connections. Pay attention to your non-verbal signals and try to be open, warm and attentive. Pay attention to non-verbal cues from others and respond accordingly to show that you are fully present and involved in the interaction.

## Have Deep Conversations:

Meaningful connections are often made through deep and meaningful conversations. Participate in discussions that go beyond superficial issues and engage with personal values, aspirations, and beliefs. Share your thoughts and actively listen to others. Outlook. These conversations create opportunities for growth, understanding and connection on a deeper level.

## Respecting Boundaries and Individuality:

Building meaningful connections requires respect for the boundaries and individuality of others. Realize that everyone has their own preferences, perspectives, and personal spaces. Respect his boundaries and avoid pushing him to share more than he is comfortable with. Appreciate and celebrate the uniqueness of each person by allowing different perspectives and experiences to enrich your relationships.

## Be Honest and Trustworthy:

Building trust is essential to meaningful relationships. Be someone others can count on and trust. Keep your commitments, keep your promises and keep your words. Show honesty and consistency in your actions and show that you can be counted on. Trust is the basis of deep bonds and fosters a sense of security and mutual respect.

## Practice Active Support:

Be there for others in need by offering support, encouragement, and listening. Celebrate their successes and help with challenges or setbacks. You actively support their development and well-being by showing that you genuinely care about their happiness and success. Their active support strengthens the bond and creates a sense of mutual support and camaraderie.

Building valuable relationships takes time, dedication, and genuine attention. By incorporating these practices into your interactions, you can build deep and fulfilling relationships that contribute to your overall attractiveness and well-being. Remember that valuable relationships are not a one-way street. So be open to others. Efforts to build a relationship with you as well.

# Chapter No. 16

# Embracing Emotional Intelligence

Using emotional intelligence is an effective way to increase your attractiveness to others. Emotional intelligence refers to the ability to recognize, understand and manage one's own emotions as well as to successfully deal with and respond to the emotions of others. These include empathy, self-awareness, self-regulation, social skills, and relationship management. Here's a broader perspective on emotional intelligence:

## Self-Awareness:

Cultivate self-awareness by paying attention to your emotions, thoughts, and reactions. Understand your strengths and weaknesses, your triggers and your values. Realize how emotions influence your behavior and decision-making. Being aware of your emotional landscape can help you better understand how it affects your interactions with others.

## Self-Regulation:

Developing the ability to effectively manage one's emotions. Practice emotion regulation techniques like deep breathing, mindfulness, and restructuring. Regulating your emotions allows you to be more thoughtful and calm in difficult situations. This self-control shows maturity and helps create a positive, harmonious environment for meaningful relationships.

## Empathy:

Empathy is the ability to understand and share the feelings of others. Practice putting yourself in another person's shoes by trying to see the world from their point of view. Actively listen, observe non-verbal cues, and acknowledge their feelings. True empathy helps build trust, fosters connection, and strengthens relationships.

## Emotion Literacy:

Developing the ability to read and write emotions by expanding emotional vocabulary and understanding the nuances of different emotions. Learn to accurately identify and articulate your emotions and recognize them in others. Increase your ability to communicate effectively and empathize with others on a deeper level.

## Active Listening:

Actively listen to others, not just what they are saying, but also the hidden emotions and needs they are expressing. Pay attention to your tone of voice, body language, and facial expressions. Show genuine interest and engagement in their stories and experiences. By practicing active listening, you show respect, acknowledge their feelings, and create a safe space for meaningful conversations.

## Conflict Resolution:

Developing conflict and disagreement skills with emotional intelligence. Handle conflicts with an emphasis on understanding, collaboration and finding win-win solutions. Practice active listening, open communication, and empathy to defuse conflict and promote healthy resolution. By using emotional intelligence to manage conflict, you build trust, strengthen bonds, and foster harmonious relationships.

## Social Skills:

Improve your social skills by improving your ability to communicate effectively, form relationships, and connect with others. Pay attention to verbal and non-verbal cues, adapt your communication style to different people and situations, and show respect and empathy when dealing with one another. Good social skills make a positive impression and make others feel comfortable and valued around you.

## Resilience:

Cultivate resilience to successfully face setbacks, challenges and adversities. Develop the ability to bounce back from setbacks and maintain a positive attitude. Resilience helps you deal with stress, remain flexible and master difficult situations. This inner strength and positivity makes you more attractive and inspiring to others.

## Emotional Support:

We provide emotional support to others by providing them with a safe space in which to express their feelings. Be compassionate, understanding, and listen without judgment. Acknowledge their feelings and offer words of encouragement and support. Emotional support strengthens your bonds and shows that you genuinely care about the well-being of others.

## Continuous Learning and Development:

Adopt a mindset of continuous learning and emotional intelligence development. Look for opportunities to develop your emotional intelligence skills through books, seminars, training, or coaching. Reflect on your experiences, get the opinions of others and work actively to improve your emotional intelligence. Demonstrating a commitment to personal growth and emotional intelligence attracts others who appreciate and appreciate these traits.

## Mindful Communication:

Practice mindful communication by being present and fully involved in the conversation. Avoid distractions and give your full attention to the person you are interacting with. Watch your words, tone of voice, and body language to ensure your communication is clear, respectful, and empathetic. Conscious communication allows for deeper understanding and connection.

## Emotional Boundaries:

Establish and respect emotional boundaries in your relationships. Recognize your emotional limits and communicate them clearly to others. Also respect the emotional boundaries set by others. Respecting emotional boundaries shows that you value, process, and prioritize the emotional well-being of yourself and others, creating a sense of security and trust.

## Emotion regulation:

Development of strategies for effective emotion regulation. Practice techniques like deep breathing, mindfulness meditation, or journaling to deal with stress, anxiety, or overwhelming emotions. When you can regulate your emotions, you are better able to respond calmly and collected, which increases your attractiveness and interpersonal interactions.

## Resolving Conflicts with Empathy:

Approach conflicts with an empathetic mindset and seek to understand the hidden emotions and perspectives of everyone involved. Practice active listening, control emotions and find common ground. By resolving conflict with empathy, you can foster understanding, resolve differences, and strengthen relationships.

## Emotional Intelligence in Leadership:

When you are in a leadership position, you use emotional intelligence to inspire and motivate others. Understand your team members' emotions and needs, provide support and encouragement, and create a positive work environment. By leading with emotional intelligence, you foster trust, loyalty, and respect in your team, making you a more attractive and effective leader.

## Non-verbal communication:

Pay attention to non-verbal signals such as facial expressions, gestures and body language. Be mindful of your non-verbal communication and try to be open, sincere, and empathetic. Also, pay attention to other people's non-verbal cues, as these can provide valuable insight into their emotional state. Effective non-verbal communication improves understanding and connection.

## Empathy for Different Experiences:

Cultivate empathy for different experiences, environments, and perspectives. Realize that individuals may have different emotional responses based on their unique life experiences. Avoid assumptions and try to understand others' feelings and points of view without judging them. Empathy for diversity promotes inclusion and strengthens relationships between different cultures and environments.

## Emotional Intelligence in Teamwork:

Use Emotional Intelligence in teamwork, promote collaboration, effective communication and understanding between team members. Encourage open dialogue, active listening, and respect for different ideas and opinions. By developing emotional intelligence in your team, you create a supportive and cohesive environment that increases productivity and success.

## Self-Reflection and Growth:

Engage in regular self-reflection to assess your emotional intelligence abilities and areas for development. Be open to feedback from others and actively seek opportunities for improvement. By constantly working to increase your emotional intelligence, you demonstrate a commitment to self-development that attracts others and helps strengthen relationships.

## Practicing Empathy Beyond Face-to-Face:

Extending empathy and emotional intelligence beyond personal relationships to broader social interactions. Practice empathy in your community, in your workplace, and when dealing with strangers. By showing empathy and compassion to people outside of your immediate environment, you help build a more empathetic and understanding society.

The acquisition of emotional intelligence is an ongoing journey of self-discovery, development and practice. By developing your emotional intelligence skills, you can deepen your relationships, effectively manage your emotions, and create a positive, engaging presence in your interactions with others.

# Chapter No. 17

# Practicing Gratitude and Mindfulness

Practicing gratitude and mindfulness can go a long way in increasing your attractiveness. These practices help develop a positive attitude, boost self-esteem, and encourage a sense of calm and presence. Here's a broader perspective on how to practice gratitude and mindfulness to increase your attractiveness:

## Gratitude Journal:

Take time each day to write down the things you're grateful for. Reflect on the positive aspects of your life, such as supportive relationships, good health, or personal achievements. Writing down your gratitude helps you focus on the positive, encourages an optimistic attitude, and makes you more attractive to others.

## Expressing Gratitude:

Take the time to express your gratitude to others. Whether it's a heartfelt thank you, a verbal appreciation, or a small act of kindness, showing gratitude to others strengthens relationships and makes a positive impression. Humans are naturally attracted to those who express gratitude and appreciate the value that others bring to their lives.

## Mindfulness Meditation:

Practice mindfulness meditation regularly to cultivate present moment awareness. Take a few minutes each day to focus on your breathing, observe your thoughts without judgment, and tune into your senses. Mindfulness meditation helps quiet the mind, reduce stress, and increase your ability to be fully present when dealing with others.

## Listening carefully:

Practice listening carefully as you speak. Give the speaker your full attention without interrupting him or formulating your answer. Listen with genuine curiosity and openness so the speaker feels heard and understood. Careful listening fosters deeper connections and shows respect and empathy.

## Mindful Eating:

Take care of your eating experience by practicing mindful eating. Slow down, savor every bite while using your senses. Pay attention to the taste, texture and aroma of your dishes. By eating mindfully, you not only increase the enjoyment of meals, but also develop a sense of gratitude for the food and for the present moment.

## Gratitude in Difficult Times:

During difficult times, consciously focus on finding something to be thankful for. It can be a lesson, an opportunity for advancement, or support for loved ones. Changing your perspective on gratitude during difficult times will help you stay resilient, attract positive energy, and inspire others with your optimism.

## Cultivate mindfulness in your daily activities:

Expand mindfulness beyond meditation by incorporating it into your daily activities. Participate in activities with full presence and attention, whether it be walking in nature, cooking meals, or spending your free time. By being fully present in every moment, you exude a sense of calm and mindfulness that others find attractive.

## Practice Self-Compassion:

Treat yourself with kindness and compassion. Recognize your strengths, forgive mistakes and take care of yourself. Cultivating self-compassion helps you develop a positive self-image and exude a sense of confidence that attracts others.

## Gratitude for others' Contribution:

Recognizing and valuing the efforts and contributions of others. Recognize the value they bring to your life, whether it be through their support, guidance, or presence. Express Your Gratitude for Others Contributions create a positive and uplifting atmosphere in your relationships.

## Conscious communication:

Pay attention to your words and their effect on others. Pause before answering, choose your words carefully, and consider your tone and body language. Mindful communication promotes understanding, minimizes misunderstandings and promotes harmonious interactions.

## Use Technology Wisely:

Be aware of your use of technology and create boundaries to avoid distractions. Set aside time for focused work or time with loved ones without electronic devices getting in the way. By being present in the moment, you show respect and create more meaningful connections.

## Gratitude for Personal Development:

Adopt an attitude of continuous development and improvement. Be grateful for opportunities for personal growth and for the lessons you learn from challenges. When you cultivate gratitude for personal growth, you show that you are open, flexible, and committed to self-improvement that others find attractive.

## Gratitude Rituals:

Establish gratitude rituals in your daily life. For example, you can start or end your day by writing down three things you are grateful for. This practice helps to focus attention on the positive aspects of life and develop a sense of gratitude. Regular gratitude rituals strengthen your positive attitude and attract others to your positive energy.

## Mindful Breathing:

Integrate mindful breathing exercises into your everyday life. Take a few moments during the day to focus on your breathing, breathing in deeply and exhaling slowly. This simple exercise helps you anchor yourself in the present moment, reduces stress, and promotes a sense of calm and focus. When you are calm and present, you exude an attractive aura of serenity.

## Gratitude for the Small Moments:

Practice gratitude for the small moments and joys in life. Admire the beauty of nature, enjoy a delicious meal or appreciate a kind gesture from a stranger. By cultivating gratitude for the small things, you develop heightened awareness and a greater ability to find joy in everyday experiences. This positive attitude is contagious and attracts others to your contagious enthusiasm.

## Mindful Body Language:

Pay attention to your body language and how it reflects your awareness and gratitude. Stand tall, adopt an open, relaxed posture, and maintain eye contact when interacting with others. These nonverbal cues convey confidence, presence, and genuine interest, making you more attractive and approachable to others.

## Gratitude in Relationships:

Practice gratitude in your relationships by regularly expressing your gratitude to loved ones. Let them know how much you appreciate and value their presence in your life. Show gratitude for their support, love, and contributions. This practice not only deepens your bonds but also strengthens the bond between you and your loved ones.

## Conscious Self-Reflection:

Engage in regular self-reflection to gain a deeper understanding of yourself and your emotions. Take some time to reflect on your thoughts, feelings, and experiences without judgment. This introspection promotes self-awareness and identifies areas for personal development. When you have a clear sense of who you are, you exude authenticity and confidence, which makes you more attractive to others.

## Gratitude in Adversity:

Cultivate gratitude even in the face of adversity. Instead of focusing on the challenges, focus on the lessons and the growth opportunities that come from them. By reframing difficulties as learning experiences, you demonstrate resilience and positivity, attractive qualities that inspire and uplift others.

## Mindful Appreciation of Others:

Practice mindful appreciation of those around you. Take the time to truly recognize and appreciate their strengths, talents, and efforts. Give sincere compliments and congratulations to lift their spirits and make them feel valued. By practicing mindful appreciation, you create a positive, supportive environment that fosters deeper connections and attracts others who appreciate your kindness and genuine appreciation.

## Gratitude for Self-Care:

Prioritize self-care and recognize the importance of taking care of your well-being. Practice gratitude for the self-care actions you take, such as B. Exercise, healthy eating, quality leisure activities and pursuing hobbies that you enjoy. By taking care of yourself, you radiate vitality and self-love, attractive qualities that inspire others to put their own well-being first.

## Conscious Presence in Social Interactions:

Be fully present in your social interactions. Put aside distractions and actively interact with the people you are with. Listen carefully, ask open-ended questions, and show interest in their stories and experiences. By practicing mindful presence, you create space for deeper connections and meaningful conversations.

## Gratitude for Personal Growth:

 Accept gratitude for your personal growth journey. Celebrate the progress you've made, no matter how small, and appreciate the effort you've made to improve. Realize that personal development is an ongoing process and that every step forward deserves gratitude. By embodying a growth mindset and expressing gratitude for your journey, you inspire others to grow and evolve.

When you incorporate gratitude and mindfulness into your life, you enrich your relationships, improve your overall well-being, and make you more attractive to others. These practices create a positive ripple effect, spreading positivity, appreciation, and genuine connection in your interactions with others.

# Chapter No. 18

# Enhancing Your Non-Verbal Communication

Improving non-verbal communication skills can go a long way in increasing your attractiveness in the eyes of others. Non-verbal signals such as body language, facial expressions, gestures and eye contact play a large role in how we perceive and interact with people. Here are some tips to help you improve your non-verbal communication and increase your attractiveness:

## Maintain good posture:

Stand or sit erect, shoulders back, and head held high. Good posture exudes confidence and can make you more attractive and approachable.

### Smile Sincerely:

A warm and sincere smile can instantly make you more attractive and likeable. Practice smiling in the mirror to ensure your smile is natural and appealing.

### Eye Contact:

Make and maintain eye contact when speaking. Show that you are attentive and interested in the other person. However, remember not to stare too much as this may make others uncomfortable.

### Use Expressive Gestures:

When speaking, use appropriate hand gestures to bring clarity and clarity to your words. However, avoid excessive or awkward movements that can obscure the message.

### Mirror:

Subtly reflects the body language of the person you are interacting with. This technique helps create contact and a sense of connection. Remember to be subtle, however, because overly accurate imitation can be viewed as insincerity or teasing.

### Provide Adequate Personal Space:

Respect personal boundaries and keep proper distance when interacting with others. Invading someone's personal space can make them feel uncomfortable and reduce your attractiveness.

### Watch your facial expressions:

Your facial expressions express emotions and can affect how others perceive you. Practice maintaining a pleasant and friendly facial expression as it can make you more approachable and attractive.

### Use a Firm Handshake:

When shaking hands, make sure your grip is firm and tight, but not too tight. A firm handshake can make a good impression and build trust.

### Dress appropriately:

The choice of clothing and hairstyle also influences non-verbal communication. Dress to suit the occasion and reflect your personal style, which will add to your overall attractiveness.

## Pay attention to the tone of your voice:

The way you speak, including tone, pitch and volume, affects how others perceive you. Look for a warm, confident, and engaging tone that conveys interest and excitement.

## Be aware of your body language:

Your body language can reveal a lot about your feelings and intentions. Maintain an open posture by keeping your arms relaxed and uncrossed, as crossed arms can signal a defensive or disinterested posture. Address your conversation partner directly and lean slightly towards them to show your commitment.

## Use the right hand gestures:

Hand gestures can be powerful communication tools. Use them consciously to emphasize your words and make your message more engaging. However, avoid excessive fuss and gestures that can distract or dilute the message.

## Control your jittery habits:

Many people engage in jittery habits like biting their nails, touching their fingers, or playing with their hair. These habits can make you appear anxious or distracted. Pay attention to them and try to replace them with more positive behaviors, such as B. by relaxing your hands or making conscious gestures.

## Develop active listening skills:

 Nonverbal communication isn't just about how you present yourself; This also includes actively listening to others. Maintain eye contact, nod occasionally to show understanding, and use facial expressions to show sympathy. These behaviors show that you are paying attention and are interested in the person speaking, which makes you more attractive as a conversationalist.

## Use Proper Touch:

Touch can be a powerful nonverbal cue, but should be used cautiously and within limits. A friendly pat on the back, handshake, or light pat on the shoulder can create a feeling of connection and warmth. Be aware of cultural norms and individual comfort levels, however, as not everyone is comfortable with physical contact.

## Be aware of your surroundings:

Your non-verbal communication needs to be adapted to different environments and situations. Pay attention to the context and adjust your body language accordingly. For example, you may be more formal and easygoing in professional settings, while being more relaxed and expressive in social situations.

## Developing Empathy and Emotional Intelligence:

Improving non-verbal communication goes hand in hand with developing empathy and emotional intelligence. Understanding and empathizing with others allows you to respond appropriately to emotions with non-verbal cues, making you more attractive as a compassionate and understanding person.

## Practice active observation:

Observe the behavior of others with strong non-verbal communication skills. Pay attention to charismatic people, speakers or actors and pay attention to their body language, facial expressions and gestures. Practice incorporating some of their techniques into your own communication style.

## Ask for feedback:

Ask a trusted friend, colleague, or mentor for feedback on your nonverbal communication. They can provide valuable information and suggestions for improvement. Be open to constructive criticism and use it to improve your skills.

## Cultivate self-confidence:

 Self-confidence is attractive and has a significant influence on non-verbal communication. Work on building your confidence by being assertive, setting and achieving goals, and stepping out of your comfort zone. As you gain confidence in yourself and your abilities, it will naturally reflect in your non-verbal cues and make you more attractive to others.

Remember that nonverbal communication is a subtle but powerful aspect of human interaction. By consciously working to improve your nonverbal signals, you can increase your attractiveness and create stronger connections with others. Practice regularly, monitor your behavior and adapt it to different situations. You will notice positive changes in the way others perceive and respond to you.

# Chapter No. 19

# Fostering Positive Relationships

Maintaining positive relationships is a key aspect of increasing attractiveness. Building meaningful relationships with others not only makes you feel better, but also makes you more attractive to those around you. Here are some strategies to help you build positive relationships and increase your overall attractiveness:

## Practice active listening:

When others are speaking, actively listen and give them your full attention. Avoid interrupting him or preparing an answer while he is still speaking. Show genuine interest by nodding, maintaining eye contact, and providing verbal and nonverbal cues that you're engaged in a conversation. Active listening fosters trust, understanding, and deepening connections with others.

## Show Empathy and Compassion:

Cultivate empathy by putting yourself in the shoes of others. shoes and try to understand her point of view and feelings. Show genuine concern for their well-being and offer your support when needed. When you show empathy and compassion, you show that you care about others, which makes you more attractive and likeable.

## Practice Effective Communication:

Communication is the foundation of any successful relationship. Try to express yourself clearly, honestly and respectfully. Avoid being overly critical or defensive and be open to opinions and different viewpoints. Effective communication creates trust, resolves conflicts and strengthens the bond with others.

## Develop Your Emotional Intelligence:

Emotional intelligence involves understanding and managing your own emotions as well as recognizing and responding to the emotions of others. Cultivate self-awareness, self-regulation, social awareness and relationship management. Emotional intelligence allows you to manage relationships more effectively, encourage positive interactions, and make you more attractive to others.

## Build Trust and Reliability:

Trust is an essential part of any healthy relationship. Be honest and keep your commitments. Show integrity by being honest, confidential and trustworthy. Reliable people are highly valued and sought after in personal and professional relationships.

## Offer support and encouragement:

Support others #039; goals and desires. Encourage, celebrate successes and provide help when needed. As a source of support and motivation, you demonstrate your willingness to invest in the well-being and success of those around you.

## Show Gratitude and Appreciation:

Express gratitude to the people in your life and recognize their contributions. Regularly show your appreciation for their efforts, kindness, and support. Gratitude promotes positive emotions and strengthens the bond between people.

## Pursue Common Interests and Activities:

Engage in activities or hobbies that align with your interests and values, and seek out others who share these passions. Participating in joint activities offers opportunities for bonding, collaboration and lasting connections.

## Forgive and Let Go of Grudges:

Holding a grudge or holding a grudge can strain relationships and decrease your attractiveness. Learn to forgive others for their mistakes and shortcomings. Practice empathy and understanding, and focus on creating positive interactions instead of worrying about past grievances.

## Be authentic and authentic:

Authenticity is very attractive because it shows that you are true to yourself and to others. Be honest in your interactions and honestly share your thoughts, feelings, and experiences. Avoid impersonating someone you are not, as this can create obstacles and hinder the development of meaningful relationships.

## Cultivate a Positive Attitude:

Maintain a positive attitude and exude positivity in your interactions. People are naturally attracted to people who exude optimism and bring positive energy to the conversation. Your positive attitude can inspire and uplift others and make you more attractive to them.

## Practice active conflict resolution:

Conflict is a natural part of any relationship, but how you deal with it can make a big difference in the outcome. Learn effective conflict resolution techniques such as active listening, expressing your feelings without blaming or judging, making compromises and finding win-win solutions. By resolving conflicts and finding solutions constructively, you demonstrate emotional maturity and the ability to rise to challenges, which makes you more attractive to others.

## Beware of Non-Verbal Cues:

As we have already seen, non-verbal communication plays a key role in relationships. When interacting, pay attention to your body language, facial expressions, and tone of voice. Make sure your nonverbal cues match your verbal communication and convey sincerity, openness, and warmth. Consistency in your nonverbal cues increases your authenticity and charm.

## Show respect and appreciation for boundaries:

Respecting personal boundaries is essential to building positive relationships. Recognize and respect the boundaries set by others, both physically and emotionally. If necessary, ask for approval and permission and take personal space into account. Respecting boundaries shows you value the autonomy of others and creates a safe and comfortable environment for deeper connections.

## Be a good team player:

Cooperation and teamwork are essential in a wide range of social and professional situations. Demonstrate the ability to work well with others by being actively involved, collaborating and respecting different opinions and viewpoints. Proving that you can be a useful and valuable team player increases your attractiveness and builds trust with your colleagues.

## Practice Active Networking:

Actively participate in networking opportunities to expand your circle of friends and build professional relationships. Attend industry events, join professional associations, or participate in community activities where you can connect with like-minded people. Networking not only broadens your contacts, but also demonstrates your proactive approach to personal and professional growth and makes you more attractive to potential employees and mentors.

## Be a Good Friend:

Cultivate strong friendships by being a loyal and supportive friend. Offer to listen, be in need, and celebrate with friends. Results. Being a reliable and trustworthy friend fosters a sense of belonging and deepens personal bonds, making you more attractive to others who value genuine friendship.

## Take Active Care of Yourself:

Taking care of your well-being is important to building positive relationships. Prioritize self-care activities that promote your physical, mental, and emotional health. By maintaining a balanced lifestyle, managing stress, and practicing self-compassion, you will become more emotionally available and able to form healthy relationships.

## Continued Investing in Personal Development:

Participate in activities that promote personal development. Expand your hobbies, acquire new skills, and acquire knowledge in areas that interest you. Personal development increases your self-confidence, enriches conversations and makes you more interesting and attractive to others.

## Be open to new experiences and perspectives:

Embrace diversity and be open to new experiences and perspectives. Take part in conversations with people from different backgrounds and cultures and actively try to understand their point of view. Accepting diversity enriches your worldview, fosters empathy, and increases your ability to make meaningful connections.

## Develop a sense of humor:

A good sense of humor is universally attractive. It lifts mood, creates positive bonds, and encourages pleasant interactions. Find joy in everyday moments, tell lighthearted jokes, and get ready to laugh at yourself. A real sense of humor makes you approachable and fun.

Remember that building positive relationships is an ongoing process that requires commitment and genuine attention. Focus on building strong bonds, practicing effective communication, and embodying qualities like empathy, respect, and authenticity. By cultivating positive relationships, you not only increase your attractiveness but also create a rewarding and supportive social network.

# Chapter No. 20

# Embracing Vulnerability and Authenticity

Accepting vulnerability and authenticity can greatly increase your attractiveness to others. When you allow yourself to be vulnerable and embrace your true self, you form deeper connections and nurture real relationships. Here's an extension on how to use vulnerability and authenticity to become more attractive:

## Understand the power of vulnerability:

Vulnerability is about opening yourself up and letting yourself be seen, heard and understood. It takes courage to express your true thoughts, feelings, and experiences, even when it's uncomfortable. Realize that vulnerability is not a weakness but a strength that enables deeper connections and authentic interactions.

## Be honest with yourself:

It starts with being honest with yourself about your feelings, desires and values. Think about your strengths, weaknesses and areas for development. Acknowledge your true self without judging or criticizing yourself. This self-confidence is the basis for accepting authenticity in dealing with others.

## Share Your Story:

Sharing your personal experiences and challenges can help you bond deeply with others. Tell your story authentically, emphasizing both triumphs and struggles. This sensitivity creates empathy and understanding and encourages others to open up.

## Express Genuine Emotions:

Allow yourself to express a wide range of emotions sincerely. Whether it's joy, sadness, excitement, or vulnerability, don't be afraid to express how you really feel. When you show genuine emotion, it encourages others to do the same, fostering deeper connections and increasing your attractiveness.

## Practice active self-acceptance:

accept your strengths, quirks and imperfections. Accept and love yourself unconditionally. When you feel good, you exude confidence and authenticity, which makes you more attractive to others.

## Avoid Impressing or Pleasing Everyone:

Being authentic means being true to yourself, even if it means displeasing everyone. You can't please everyone, so focus on staying true to your values and beliefs. People are attracted to people who don't compromise.

## Be open to the vulnerability of others:

Encourage others around you and create a safe space for sensitivity. Listen without judgment, offer support, and validate their experiences. When you show acceptance and compassion for other sensitivities, they are more likely to retaliate, deepen the relationship, and be attracted to one another.

## Cultivating Self-Compassion:

Treat yourself with kindness and compassion. Be understanding and forgive your mistakes and failures. When you practice self-compassion, you can be more authentic with others because you're not constantly striving for validation or perfection.

## Practice Active and Empathetic Listening:

Really listen to others with an open mind and heart. Pay attention to their words, emotions and body language. Show genuine interest in understanding their point of view and experiences. Active, empathetic listening creates a safe space for authentic conversations and strengthens relationships.

## Being comfortable in stillness:

Accepting your sensitivity also means being comfortable in moments of stillness. Allow yourself to reflect and connect more deeply without feeling the need to fill each moment with words. Comfortable silence can promote intimacy and create an atmosphere of trust and understanding.

## Seek Meaningful Relationships:

Focus on maintaining good relationships rather than trying to impress or attract many people. Invest your time and energy in building deep and meaningful relationships with people who appreciate and value your authenticity.

## Embrace growth and learning:

Authenticity does not mean stagnation. Keep developing, learning and growing. Be open to new experiences, perspectives and ideas. By embracing growth and learning, you can constantly deepen your authenticity and attractiveness.

## Challenging Society's Expectations:

Society often sets strict expectations and standards for our behavior and presentation. Accepting vulnerability and authenticity means challenging these social norms and accepting your true self, even when it defies conventional expectations. By freeing yourself from social pressures, you inspire others to do the same and create a more open and tolerant environment.

## Practice Self-Reflection:

Engage in self-reflection regularly to understand your thoughts, feelings, and motivations. Take the time to question your fears, insecurities and limiting beliefs. This introspection allows you to discover your authentic self and identify areas where you can be most sensitive and true to yourself.

## Get Out of Your Comfort Zone:

In order to accept your weaknesses, you often have to get out of your comfort zone and take risks. This may include starting difficult conversations, looking for new opportunities, or sharing personal stories that make you feel vulnerable. By accepting discomfort and taking calculated risks, you display courage and authenticity, very attractive qualities.

## Be Open to Feedback:

Actively seek feedback from trusted individuals who can provide honest and constructive ideas. Accepting vulnerability means being open to feedback, even though it can be difficult to hear. Use feedback as an opportunity for personal growth and improvement so you can become a more authentic and engaged person.

## Celebrate Your Uniqueness:

Appreciate and celebrate the aspects of yourself that make you unique. Whether it's your quirks, talents, or unconventional interests, owning and expressing your uniqueness can really make you stand out from the crowd. By accepting and sharing your individuality, you attract others who value and are attracted to your true self.

## Express yourself:

Find creative ways to express yourself that match your passions and interests. This can be through art, writing, music or any other form of creative expression. Participating in activities that allow you to express yourself authentically encourages self-discovery and increases attractiveness by flaunting your passion and authenticity.

## Build a support network:

Surround yourself with people who encourage and support your vulnerability and authenticity. Look for like-minded people who appreciate and appreciate authentic relationships. A strong support network provides validation and acceptance, so you can address vulnerabilities with greater confidence.

## Practicing Self-Care and Self-Compassion:

Self-care through self-care and self-compassion practices is critical to overcoming vulnerability. Offer yourself kindness, understanding, and forgiveness. Practice self-care activities that replenish your energy and encourage self-acceptance. When you put your wellbeing first, you exude authenticity and attract others who value self-love and compassion.

## Share Your Passions and Interests:

Share your true passions and interests with others. Participate in conversations and activities that match your true passions. When you express enthusiasm and authenticity in the things you enjoy, it becomes contagious and attractive to others who appreciate your genuine enthusiasm.

## Accepting Imperfections:

Coming to terms with weaknesses means accepting and accepting your own imperfections. Realize that nobody is perfect and that imperfections make us human. Accepting and confronting your flaws not only promotes self-acceptance but also makes others around you feel more comfortable being themselves.

Remember that acceptance of sensitivity and authenticity is an ongoing process that requires self-awareness, self-acceptance and constant evolution. By accepting vulnerability, you create deeper connections, attract like-minded people, and nurture a more fulfilling and attractive life.

# Chapter No. 21

# Cultivating Kindness and Empathy

Cultivating kindness and empathy is a great way to increase your attractiveness as a person. Even if your outward appearance initially draws the attention of others, your inner qualities really make a lasting impression and draw people to you. Here are some ways that cultivating kindness and empathy can make you more attractive:

**Real Connection:**

Kindness and empathy allow you to connect more deeply with others. When you genuinely care about people's well-being, you inspire a sense of trust and understanding. It can lead to more meaningful relationships and connections, and make you more attractive as a friend, partner, or colleague.

## Positive Energy:

Kindness and empathy radiate positive energy. When you genuinely care about others and treat them with compassion, you create an uplifting atmosphere that people are naturally drawn to. Your positive attitude and caring attitude can make you a magnet for social interactions and create a pleasant atmosphere wherever you go.

## Emotional Support:

Empathy allows you to understand and share the emotions of others. By providing a supportive shoulder to lean on, you become someone others can rely on in difficult times. Your ability to listen, comfort, and guide makes you more attractive as a confidant and source of emotional support.

## Conflict Resolution:

Kindness and empathy are key to resolving conflicts and building harmonious relationships. When disagreements arise, you can approach the situation with understanding and compassion, and seek a solution that satisfies everyone involved. Your ability to resolve conflicts peacefully demonstrates maturity and emotional intelligence that make you more attractive to others.

## Altruism:

Acting kindly and showing compassion to those in need shows your unselfishness and generosity. Whether you volunteer, support charities, or just help, your commitment to making a positive difference in the lives of others demonstrates attractive qualities such as empathy, compassion, and a sense of social responsibility.

## Better Communication:

Kindness and empathy improve your communication skills. By actively listening and showing genuine interest in others, you can build stronger connections and understand different viewpoints. Effective communication is a very attractive trait because it promotes understanding, reduces misunderstandings, and promotes healthier relationships.

## Personal Growth:

Cultivating kindness and empathy allows you to continually grow as an individual. It encourages self-reflection and self-improvement, leading to greater emotional intelligence and a broader outlook on life. People are often attracted to people who demonstrate personal growth and actively work on themselves, which makes you more attractive in a personal and professional setting.

## Practice Self-Compassion:

It's important to develop kindness and empathy toward yourself before projecting it onto others. Treat yourself with compassion and understand that everyone makes mistakes and faces challenges. By cultivating self-compassion, you will unlock a sense of inner satisfaction and confidence, which in turn will make you more attractive to others.

## Active Listening:

Truly listening to others is an effective way to show empathy. Practice active listening by giving your full attention, maintaining eye contact and not interrupting. Show genuine interest in what others have to say and ask open-ended questions to encourage them to say more. It encourages deeper connections and shows you value their thoughts and feelings.

## Imagine others' Boots:

Empathy is about understanding and sharing the feelings of others. When you interact with someone, try to imagine their perspective, experiences, and feelings. This empathetic approach helps you respond with sensitivity and consideration, and make others feel heard and understood. Acknowledging your feelings can go a long way in building trust and relationships.

## Practice casual acts of kindness:

Small acts of kindness can have a significant impact on others and make you more attractive. These activities may include opening a door for someone, giving a sincere compliment, or helping someone with a task. In your daily life, look for ways to spread positivity and make someone's day a little bit better.

## Cultivating Gratitude:

Gratitude helps cultivate kindness and empathy by encouraging a positive attitude. Take time each day to reflect on the things you're grateful for, whether it's the people in your life, your accomplishments, or simple joys. This change in mindset can increase your overall happiness, make you more attractive while exuding a sense of accomplishment and appreciation.

**Volunteering and Giving Back:** Getting involved in community work or volunteering for a cause you care about is a great way to show kindness and empathy. Offer your time and skills to help those in need, whether it's a local animal shelter, hospital, or charity. Giving back not only benefits those you help, but also strengthens your empathy and sense of purpose, and makes you more attractive as a compassionate and socially conscious person.

## Practice Emotion Regulation:

Being kind and empathetic requires managing your emotions effectively. Develop emotional intelligence by recognizing and understanding your feelings and reactions. This self-awareness enables you to react calmly and empathetically to others, even in difficult situations. People are naturally attracted to people who can handle their emotions with grace and compassion.

## Do perspective exercises:

Build your empathy by participating in perspective exercises. Put yourself in the other person's shoes, given their backgrounds, experiences and challenges.

Remember that developing kindness and empathy is an ongoing journey that requires constant effort. By incorporating these practices into your daily life, you not only improve your well-being, you also become a magnet for positive relationships and experiences. Your sincere caring and understanding will make you more attractive to others, foster deep connections, and enrich your personal and professional life.

# Chapter No. 22

# Embracing Imperfections and Self-Compassion

Accepting imperfections and practicing self-compassion is a powerful way to increase your attractiveness as an individual. It's about accepting and loving yourself for who you are, with flaws and everything that can have a transformative effect on your confidence and the way others see you. Here are some ways to accept your imperfections and practice self-compassion to become more attractive:

**Authenticity:**

Accepting your imperfections allows you to be authentic and honest. When you are comfortable with who you are, including your flaws and weaknesses, you exude a sense of trust and authenticity that is extremely appealing to others. People appreciate people who don't compromise and you are more likely to be attracted to their unique qualities.

## Confidence:

Accepting imperfections helps develop strong self-confidence. Instead of constantly striving for perfection or comparing yourself to unrealistic standards, realize that everyone has flaws and doesn't define your worth. This confidence exudes attractiveness and attraction, attracting others with its positive energy and confidence.

## Affinity:

By accepting imperfections, you become more identifiable with others. Nobody is perfect, and when you openly admit your imperfections, you create a sense of connection with other people who may be struggling with similar insecurities. Your vulnerability and self-acceptance make you accessible and available, which fosters deeper and more meaningful connections.

## Emotional Resilience:

Accepting imperfections is closely related to self-compassion, which means treating yourself with kindness and understanding in times of struggle or defeat. This practice increases your emotional resilience and your ability to recover from setbacks. People are often drawn to those who can meet challenges with grace and compassion, as this inspires them to do the same.

## Positive Self-Image:

Embracing Imperfections and Practicing Self-Compassion Cultivate a positive self-image. Instead of focusing on perceived flaws, focus on your unique strengths, accomplishments, and qualities. This positive self-esteem increases confidence and attractiveness because it allows you to present yourself in a more positive and authentic light.

## Healthy Relationships:

Accepting imperfections and practicing self-compassion also have profound effects on your relationships. When you fully accept yourself, you are more likely to form healthy and supportive relationships. You are less likely to tolerate toxic behavior or settle for less than you deserve. Your self-compassion sets the standard for how others should treat you and leads to more fulfilling and respectful relationships.

## Emotional Wellbeing:

When you accept your imperfections and practice self-compassion, your overall emotional wellbeing improves greatly. By being kind to yourself, you develop a sense of inner peace and contentment. This positive emotional state is attractive to others because it creates an uplifting and harmonious presence that people naturally strive for.

## Inspire Others:

As you accept your imperfections and practice self-compassion, you become an inspiration to others. Her ability to face challenges and setbacks with grace and self-acceptance is a striking example of this. By being kind to yourself, you encourage others to accept their imperfections and develop self-compassion, creating a positive impact that transcends yourself.

## Authenticity and Vulnerability:

Accepting imperfections allows you to show others your true self, thereby empowering authenticity and vulnerability. When you speak openly about your mistakes and insecurities, you create a safe space where others can do the same. This authenticity deepens bonds and attracts people who value authentic and meaningful relationships.

## Empathy and Understanding:

To practice self-compassion, one must treat oneself with the same kindness and understanding that one would treat others. When you develop empathy for yourself, you also become more empathetic towards others. Your ability to understand and empathize with the difficulties and imperfections of others makes you an attractive and compassionate person.

## Spiritual Growth:

Accepting Imperfections and Practicing Self-Compassion Cultivate a growth mindset. Don't look at mistakes or setbacks as failures, but as opportunities to learn and grow. This mindset attracts others who are equally motivated to learn, grow, and overcome challenges, leading to more fulfilling and vibrant relationships.

## Avoid Comparisons:

Accepting imperfections means giving up the desire to compare yourself to others. Instead of striving for an unrealistic ideal, focus on your progress and celebrate your unique qualities. This changed mindset not only increases your self-esteem, but also allows you to appreciate and support the achievements of others, making you a truly supportive and attractive person.

## Emotional Intelligence:

Self-compassion increases emotional intelligence, which is an attractive trait in any relationship. By listening to your feelings and being kind to yourself, you will be better able to understand and respond to the feelings of others. This emotional intelligence allows for deeper connections and effective communication, making you more attractive in human interactions.

## Boundaries and Self-Esteem:

Accepting imperfections and practicing self-compassion can help you set healthy boundaries and prioritize self-esteem. You become more discerning about choosing relationships and situations that align with your values and well-being. This confidence and self-care is very appealing because it shows strong self-esteem and personal empowerment.

## Inner Happiness and Fulfillment:

Accepting imperfections and practicing self-compassion promotes inner happiness and contentment. Instead of striving for external validation, find fulfillment within. This radiant joy and contentment makes you naturally attractive and attracts others to your positive energy and optimism.

## Inspire others to be authentic:

By accepting imperfections and practicing self-compassion, you inspire others to do the same. Your willingness to be vulnerable and accept yourself sets an example for others to accept your imperfections and practice self-compassion. This ripple effect can create a supportive and caring environment where everyone feels safe to be themselves.

Remember that accepting imperfections and practicing self-compassion is an ongoing process that requires patience and self-reflection. On this journey, be kind to yourself and remember that true attractiveness comes from within. By cultivating self-compassion, you can make real connections, inspire others, and form more indulgent, loving relationships with yourself and those around you.

# Chapter No. 23

# Overcoming Self-Doubt and Limiting Beliefs

The feeling of attractiveness and self-confidence depends not only on external factors, but also on the inner mindset and self-perception. Overcoming self-doubt and limiting beliefs can go a long way in making you more attractive. Here are some strategies that can help you in this process:

## Challenge Negative Thoughts:

Identify and challenge negative thoughts that contribute to insecurity or reduce beliefs about your attractiveness. Replace them with positive, realistic affirmations. For example, instead of thinking "I'm unattractive," replace it with "I have unique qualities that make me attractive.""

## Accept yourself:

Understand that attractiveness is subjective and varies from person to person. Focus on accepting and valuing yourself for who you are, including your looks, personality, and achievements. Celebrate your strengths and work to improve in the areas that matter to you.

## Take Care of Yourself:

Taking care of yourself physically, emotionally, and spiritually can increase your confidence and overall attractiveness. Develop a routine that includes regular exercise, a healthy diet, adequate sleep, personal hygiene, and clothing that makes you feel good.

## Surround yourself with positivity:

Surround yourself with supportive and positive influences such as friends, family, or mentors who will encourage you and help you build your self-esteem. Limit your exposure to negative or toxic people who depress you or increase your insecurity.

## Set achievable goals:

Setting goals and achieving them can boost your confidence. Break larger goals down into smaller, achievable steps and celebrate your progress along the way. This process can help you realize your potential and create a sense of accomplishment.

## Cultivating Compassion:

Treat yourself with kindness and understanding. Accept the fact that everyone has imperfections and flaws and learn to forgive yourself for them. Practice self-compassion by speaking to yourself in nurturing and encouraging ways, just as you would a friend in a similar situation.

## Build a Positive Self-Image:

Improve your self-image by focusing on your positive qualities. Make a list of your strengths, talents, and achievements. Remind yourself of these qualities regularly to counteract negative self-perceptions.

## Discover Your Personal Interests:

Engaging in activities and hobbies that bring you joy and fulfillment can boost your self-confidence. Pursue your passions, learn new skills, and invest time in activities that make you confident and attractive.

## Seek professional help as needed:

If you continue to suffer from self-doubt and limiting beliefs, consider seeking the advice of a therapist or counselor. They can help you identify and solve underlying problems and provide strategies for overcoming them successfully.

## Practice Empowerment:

Take control of your life and actively make choices that align with your values and desires. When you feel empowered, it has a positive effect on your image and attractiveness. Set boundaries, be confident, and make decisions that put your well-being and happiness first.

## Cultivate a growth mindset:

Trust that you can grow and improve over time. The growth mentality allows you to see challenges as opportunities for growth rather than indicators of your limitations. By committing to continuous learning and seeing failure as a stepping stone, you can increase your confidence and attractiveness.

## Focus on Inner Qualities:

Attractiveness isn't just about outward appearance, it's also about inner qualities. Develop positive character traits such as kindness, empathy, humor and trust. These traits exude attractiveness and create genuine bonds with others.

## Practicing Gratitude:

Cultivating gratitude can shift your focus from insecurities and limiting beliefs to recognizing the positive aspects of your life. Regularly express gratitude for your strengths, achievements, and the support you receive from others. This practice can increase self-esteem and overall attractiveness.

## Start a Positive Internal Conversation:

Be careful how you talk to yourself. Replace self-critical and negative self-talk with positive and encouraging affirmations. Treat yourself with kindness, compassion and understanding. Think about your worth and your worth as a person.

## Get Out of Your Comfort Zone:

Stepping out of your comfort zone allows you to grow and develop new skills and experiences. Challenge yourself to try new things, take calculated risks and seize opportunities for personal growth. Every time you step out of your comfort zone, you gain confidence and attractiveness.

## Be inspired by others:

Surround yourself with models and people who inspire you. Look for people who have overcome doubts and limiting beliefs and found success in life. Learn from their travels, seek advice whenever possible, and let their stories motivate you to overcome your challenges.

## Practice mindfulness and self-reflection:

Engage in mindfulness practices such as meditation or journaling to develop self-awareness and better understand your thoughts and feelings. When you understand the causes of insecurity and limiting beliefs, you can deal with them more effectively and develop a more positive self-perception.

## Take Care of Your Physical Health:

While attractiveness isn't just about looks, taking care of your physical health can have a positive impact on your confidence and overall well-being. Exercise regularly, eat a balanced diet and get enough sleep. These practices can boost your energy levels, improve your mood, and increase your attractiveness.

Remember that overcoming doubts and limiting beliefs is a journey that will take time and effort. Be patient with yourself and celebrate the small victories along the way. By consistently implementing these strategies, you can develop a positive self-image, increase your self-esteem and radiate attractiveness from within.

# Chapter No. 24

# Unleashing Your Creative Expression

Unleashing creative expression can be a powerful tool for increasing attractiveness. When you let your creativity run wild, you foster a sense of authenticity, passion, and uniqueness that can be very appealing to others. Here are some ways to expand on the idea of using creative expression to make yourself more attractive:

**Explore Your Creative Possibilities:**

Explore different creative ways to find what appeals to you. This can be painting, writing, dancing, playing a musical instrument, cooking, photography or any other form of artistic expression. Experiment with different activities until you find ones that spark your passion and allow you to express yourself authentically.

## Adopt your own unique style:

Use your creativity to develop your own style. Experiment with different fashions, hairstyles, accessories and makeup to find what gives you confidence and reflects your personality. Don't be afraid to be bold and express yourself through your looks. When you feel comfortable and authentic in your style, your attractiveness increases.

## Express yourself through body language:

Your body language plays a big part in how others perceive you. Use creative expression to convey your emotions, confidence and energy through your body. Practice open and relaxed postures, make purposeful gestures and use your body to make yourself understood. Participating in activities like dance or theater can help you express yourself better physically.

## Embrace Creativity in Social Interactions:

Incorporate creativity into your social interactions by engaging in meaningful conversations, storytelling, and active listening. Develop your communication skills to effectively express your thoughts and feelings. Use your creativity to find interesting and unique ways to connect with others, such as sharing stories, asking thought-provoking questions, or using humor and wit.

## Create a Positive and Inspiring Environment:

Use your creative abilities to create an environment that inspires and cheers you and those around you up. Design your living space to reflect your personality and create a welcoming atmosphere. Surround yourself with art, colors and objects that inspire you. By creating a positive environment, you exude attractiveness and attract others who will appreciate your creative energy.

## Collaborate with others:

Participating in collaborative creative projects can help you connect with like-minded people and develop your creative skills. Join art classes, writing groups, or drama workshops where you can collaborate and learn from the unique perspective of others. This partnership not only sparks your creativity, but also creates opportunities to build relationships and attract people who appreciate your creative expression.

## Accept imperfection and take risks:

Creativity thrives when you let go of the fear of failure and accept imperfection. Allow yourself to take risks, try new things and learn from your mistakes. Understand that creativity is a process and it's okay to make mistakes or create imperfect work. Accepting imperfection allows one to express oneself freely and authentically, which is very attractive.

## Get Inspiration from Different Sources:

Broaden your creative horizons by getting inspiration from different sources. Explore different art forms, cultures, music genres, literature and other forms of creative expression. This confrontation with diverse influences broadens your perspective, promotes your creativity and broadens your perspective. and allows you to bring a unique blend of ideas and inspiration to your creative endeavors.

## Practice Self-Reflection and Introspection:

 Creative expression can be a powerful tool for self-reflection and introspection. Use your creative activities as an opportunity to explore your emotions, thoughts, and experiences. This process can increase your self-awareness, help you understand better, and contribute to your personal development by making you more attractive and showing depth and insight.

## Share Your Creative Journey:

Don't be afraid to share your creative journey with others. Whether you're exhibiting artwork, performing on stage, sharing your lyrics, or any other form of creative expression, sharing your passion and creativity can be very exciting. It allows others to see your authentic self and connect with your unique perspective.

## Using Storytelling to Engage Others:

Storytelling is a powerful form of creative expression that can engage and captivate others. Develop your storytelling skills by sharing personal anecdotes, telling stories, or making up fictional stories. This skill can make you an interesting and charismatic communicator who gets the attention of others.

## Participate in Creative Problem Solving:

Creative expression goes beyond traditional artistic pursuits. Apply your creativity to problem solving in various aspects of your life. Think outside the box, generate innovative ideas and tackle challenges with a creative spirit. This ability to find unique solutions and be creative in problem solving can be very attractive to others.

## Discover the connection between creativity and self-confidence:

Creative expression can increase your self-confidence. As you engage creatively, you develop a sense of mastery and accomplishment, which translates into greater self-confidence. The confidence gained through creative self-expression can have a positive impact on your overall attractiveness and the way you interact with others.

## Embodiment Passion and Excitement:

When you express yourself creatively, you channel your passion and enthusiasm into your work. Let your love of creative pursuits shine through in your actions and interactions. Enthusiasm is contagious and can attract others who appreciate your zest for life and creative energy.

## Take a Creative Workshop or Class:

Attending a creative workshop or class is a great way to learn new techniques, improve your skills, and connect with other creative people. These environments provide opportunities for growth, inspiration and networking. By immersing yourself in a community of like-minded people, you'll develop your creative skills and attract others who share your passion.

## Use Creativity to Develop a Sense of Fun:

Incorporate fun into your creative expression. The game inspires joy, encourages exploration and ensures light-hearted interactions. Whether you're improvising, having artistic fun, or just adding humor to your conversations, a playful approach can make you more engaging and fun to socialize.

## Allow vulnerability in your creative expression:

Authentic and sensitive expression through creativity can be incredibly appealing. Don't be afraid to reveal your true self, share your personal experiences and express your feelings through your creative activities. Such an opening can create deep connections with others and foster a sense of trust and authenticity.

## Constantly Foster Your Creativity:

Creativity is not a finite resource, but a skill that can be nurtured and developed. Spend time regularly on creative pursuits, discovering new techniques and looking for inspiration. By devoting yourself to continuous development and improvement, you increase your creative abilities and become more attractive as you grow as an individual.

## Supporting and appreciating others #039; Creativity:

Shows genuine interest and appreciation for the creative expression of others. By supporting and encouraging other artists, musicians, writers or creators in any field, you create a positive atmosphere of collaboration. This mindset of celebrating and appreciating the creativity of others makes you more attractive because it shows your generosity and appreciation for the creative spirit.

## Master an experimental and inquiring mindset:

Creativity thrives when you allow yourself to explore uncharted territory and experiment. Don't be afraid to try new techniques, combine different art forms or step out of your comfort zone. This experimental and exploratory mindset not only boosts your creativity but also makes you more interesting and attractive to others.

Remember that creative expression is deeply personal and the most attractive form of creativity is that which springs from your authentic self. Embrace your unique perspective, express yourself with confidence, and share your creative journey with others. This will increase your attractiveness and connection to people who value and align with your creative spirit.

# Chapter No. 25

# Embracing Change and Personal Growth

Accepting change and self-development can go a long way in increasing your attractiveness. When you actively seek personal growth and embrace change, you display qualities that others find extremely attractive, such as: B. Resilience, adaptability and a growth mentality. Here are some ways to develop the idea of embracing change and personal advancement to increase your attractiveness:

## Foster a growth mindset:

Adopting a growth mindset is essential to personal growth and attracting others. You believe that your skills and intelligence can be developed through dedication and effort. Focus on learning from challenges and setbacks and see them as opportunities for growth, not failures. This mindset not only increases your attractiveness but also inspires others to grow with you.

## Set goals and work towards them:

Setting meaningful goals and striving to achieve them is an attractive trait. Shows ambition, determination and a desire to improve. Set short- and long-term goals, break them down into actionable steps, and track your progress. As you move closer to your goals, you exude confidence and inspire others with your commitment to personal growth.

## Deal with your discomfort and get out of your comfort zone:

Growth and transformation often take place outside of your comfort zone. Challenge yourself to try new things, take calculated risks and deal with situations that might feel uncomfortable at first. By accepting discomfort, you develop resilience and adaptability—traits that make you more attractive to others.

## Cultivate the habit of self-reflection:

regularly reflect on your thoughts, actions and experiences. Engage in introspection to become self-aware and better understand your strengths, weaknesses, and areas for improvement. This self-reflection allows you to make conscious changes and refine your behavior, making you more attractive as you show your commitment to personal growth.

## Continuous learning and the acquisition of new skills:

Lifelong learning is a central aspect of personal development. Participate in activities that expand your knowledge and skills. Take courses, read books, attend workshops or use online learning platforms to gain new knowledge and develop new skills. Broadening your horizons makes you more interesting and attractive to others.

## Accept change as an opportunity for growth:

Change is inevitable in life and accepting it can lead to personal growth and increase attractiveness. Instead of resisting change, see it as an opportunity to learn, adapt and grow.

When you embrace change with a positive attitude, you can gracefully navigate life's changes and inspire others with your resilience.

## Soliciting feedback and constructive criticism:

Proactively seek feedback from trusted individuals such as mentors, friends, or co-workers. Feedback provides valuable insight into areas where you can improve and grow. Be open to constructive criticism and use it as a catalyst for personal development. By showing a willingness to learn and develop, you become more attractive to others.

## Develop Resilience and Recover from Setbacks:

Resilience is an attractive trait that demonstrates your ability to recover from adversity. When you face setbacks or setbacks, see them as learning opportunities and use them to build your resilience. Focus on finding solutions, learning and growing from experiences. Your resilience and ability to meet challenges with grace make you more attractive and inspiring to others.

## Developing Emotional Intelligence:

Emotional intelligence, which involves understanding and managing emotions, is an important aspect of personal development. Develop confidence, empathy and effective communication skills. By understanding your emotions and adjusting to the emotions of others, you make meaningful connections and increase your attractiveness.

## Surround yourself with people who develop:

Surround yourself with people who inspire and support you in your personal development. Look for relationships and communities that value personal growth and encourage you to become the best version of yourself. A growth-friendly environment can significantly increase your attractiveness and provide you with valuable support throughout the process.

## Take Care of Yourself and Your Wellbeing:

Taking care of your physical, mental, and emotional wellbeing is critical to personal development and attractiveness. Prioritize self-care activities like exercise, good nutrition, good sleep, and stress management. When you put your wellbeing first, you exude confidence and exude a positive attitude that makes you more attractive to others.

## Share Your Personal Development Journey:

Be open and transparent about your personal development journey with others. Share your experiences, lessons learned and steps you are taking to improve. This vulnerability and authenticity not only allows you to identify with yourself, but also inspires and motivates others to embark on their own journey of personal growth.

## Developing a Positive Attitude:

Developing a positive attitude is key to accepting change and personal growth. Focus on gratitude, optimism and self-confidence. Train your mind to see opportunities in challenges, turn failures into new experiences, and approach new situations with a positive attitude. A positive attitude not only increases your attractiveness but also attracts others who are attracted to your positive energy.

## Practice Self-Compassion:

On the path to personal growth, it is important to practice self-compassion. Be kind and understanding with yourself, especially in times of difficulty or failure. Treat yourself with the same compassion and care that you would treat a dear friend. By cultivating self-compassion, you strengthen your resilience, strengthen your self-esteem and radiate a confident and attractive aura.

## Take a holistic approach to personal development:

Personal development encompasses various aspects of your life, including physical, emotional, mental, and spiritual well-being. Take a holistic approach by nurturing all of these areas. Engage in activities that promote balance and alignment, such as regular exercise, mindfulness or meditation practices, hobbies you enjoy, and nurturing meaningful relationships.

## Encourage adaptability and openness:

Accepting change requires adaptability and openness to new experiences, ideas and perspectives. Challenge yourself to leave your comfort zone and explore new territory. Contact with other people and cultures, trying out new activities and looking for other perspectives broaden your horizons, increase your personal development and make you more attractive through openness.

## Taking responsibility for your own development:

Personal development is a personal journey and requires that you take responsibility for your own development. Realize that you have the power to shape your life and make informed decisions that will contribute to your growth. Take responsibility for your actions, decisions, and the direction of your life. By demonstrating your drive and proactive approach to personal development, you will be more attractive to others who appreciate your drive and responsibility.

## Seeks Challenges and Learning Opportunities:

Actively seeks challenges and learning opportunities that take you beyond your comfort zone. Participate in activities that develop your skills and promote personal growth. This may include taking on new projects at work, enrolling in classes or seminars, or pursuing hobbies that require you to develop new skills. By tackling these challenges, you demonstrate your drive to grow and inspire others with your commitment to self-improvement.

## Foster your resilience by taking care of yourself:

 Self-care is key to building resilience and supporting personal growth. Prioritize activities that promote your well-being, give you energy and encourage self-reflection. Do exercises like journaling, meditation, spend time in nature, or take part in creative outings? By prioritizing self-care, you strengthen your ability to deal with change, recover from setbacks, and maintain a positive, engaged presence.

## Share your developmental journey with others:

Share your personal developmental journey with authenticity and sensitivity. Discuss openly the challenges you faced, the lessons you learned, and the changes you experienced. By sharing your story, you create a sense of connection and inspire others to embark on their own development journey. Authenticity and vulnerability are very attractive traits that encourage meaningful connections.

Remember that personal development is a lifelong process and it is important to follow the path and not just focus on the goal. Accepting change, seeking opportunities for personal growth, and caring about your well-being all contribute to your attractiveness as an individual. By constantly evolving and growing, you not only improve your life, but you also inspire and attract others who are attracted to your growth mindset.

# Chapter No. 26

# Embodying Confidence and Assertiveness

Embodying confidence and assertiveness can significantly increase your attractiveness. Confidence is an attractive trait that signals confidence and inner strength, while assertiveness allows you to communicate your needs and boundaries effectively. Here are some ways to develop the embodiment of confidence and assertiveness to become more attractive:

## Developing Self-Confidence:

Self-confidence is the foundation of confidence and assertiveness. Take the time to understand your strengths, values, and beliefs. Identify your areas of development and work to improve them. By gaining a deep understanding of yourself, you can convey an authentic and confident image of yourself to others.

## Maintain Positive Self-Talk:

Pay attention to your self-talk and question any negative or self-limiting thoughts. Replace them with positive affirmations and uplifting affirmations. By having a positive inner conversation, you build self-confidence and instill confidence in those around you.

## Adopt the right posture and body language:

Your body language plays a crucial role in how others perceive you. Stand tall, maintain good posture, and maintain eye contact when interacting with others. Use open, expansive gestures to convey confidence and assertiveness. A confident posture can make you more attractive and approachable.

## Setting and Enforcing Healthy Boundaries:

Setting and enforcing personal boundaries is an important aspect of assertiveness. Be clear about your boundaries and expectations with others and make sure you stick to them. When you respect your boundaries, you demonstrate self-esteem and earn the respect of others.

## Practice Effective Communication:

Develop strong communication skills to express your thoughts, feelings, and needs clearly and confidently. Use the "I" statement to express yourself without becoming overly aggressive or passive. Active listening is also essential for effective communication as it shows respect for others. Outlook. Effective communication creates trust and increases your attractiveness in social and professional contacts.

## Celebrate your successes:

Recognize and celebrate your big and small successes. Recognize your skills and the progress you've made in your personal and professional journey. Celebrating success builds self-confidence and releases positive energy that attracts others.

## Take calculated risks:

Stepping out of your comfort zone and taking calculated risks can boost your confidence and security. Challenge yourself to try new things, take on new responsibilities and take advantage of development opportunities. Even if the outcome isn't always perfect, taking risks shows your confidence in your abilities and makes you more attractive to others.

## See failure as a learning opportunity:

Failure is a natural part of personal development. Instead of getting discouraged by failure, look at it as an opportunity to learn. Analyze what went wrong, learn valuable insights and apply this information to your future projects. Your ability to overcome setbacks with resilience and determination shows your confidence and makes you more attractive.

## Take care of your physical well-being:

Self-care measures such as regular exercise, a healthy diet and sufficient rest contribute to well-being and self-confidence. Taking care of your physical health gives you energy, improves your mood and makes you look good. When you feel physically good, it has a positive effect on your confidence and attractiveness.

## Self-Acceptance and Self-Love:

Self-acceptance and the practice of self-love are key to embodying confidence and assertiveness. Appreciate your strengths, accept your imperfections, and love yourself unconditionally. When you truly love and accept yourself, it shines from within and makes you more attractive to others.

## Practice Assertive Decision-Making:

Assertive decision-making is about making decisions based on your values, desires, and priorities. Avoid giving in to outside pressure or seeking validation from others. Trust your instincts and make decisions with confidence. Assertive decision-making demonstrates your independence and confidence, which makes you more attractive.

## Seeks opportunities for personal and professional growth:

Constantly seeks opportunities for personal and professional growth. Gain new knowledge, develop new skills and challenge yourself to reach new heights. A growth mindset demonstrates ambition, determination, and confidence that make you more attractive to others.

## Self-Care and Self-Improvement:

Prioritize self-care practices that promote your well-being and boost your self-confidence. This may include activities such as practicing mindfulness or meditation, pursuing a hobby you enjoy, indulging in self-care rituals, or engaging in activities that promote relaxation and stress reduction. Investing the time and energy to take care of yourself is a clear signal that you value your needs and put them first, which makes you more attractive to others.

## Develop Strong Self-Esteem:

Take the time to discover your values, your passions, and your interests. Realize who you are in your heart and what you stand for. When you have strong self-esteem, you are more grounded and confident in expressing your thoughts, opinions, and desires. This authenticity and self-confidence makes you attractive and appealing to others.

## Cultivate Resilience and Adaptability:

Life is full of challenges and setbacks, but developing resilience and adaptability allows you to face them with confidence. See adversity as an opportunity to grow and learn. When you face, learn from, and emerge stronger from difficult situations, you demonstrate resilience and adaptability—attractive qualities that inspire others.

## Surround yourself with favorable and positive influences:

The company you work with plays an important role in your self-esteem and assertiveness. Surround yourself with encouraging, positive and uplifting people who support your development and believe in your abilities. Your presence and encouragement will boost your confidence and help you embody assertiveness more naturally.

## Practice Empowerment:

Take control of your life and actively make choices that align with your goals and values. Avoid asking others for confirmation or approval before taking action. Trust your abilities and your intuition and empower yourself to make the decisions that are in your best interest. Empowerment demonstrates confidence and assertiveness, which makes you more attractive to those who value confident people.

## Cultivate a Growth Mentality:

Adopt a mindset of continuous learning and growth. See challenges as opportunities for growth, not obstacles. Accept the idea that you can always improve and develop new skills. Not only does this attitude boost your self-confidence, but it also makes you more flexible and open to change—traits that others find very attractive.

## Practice Assertive Body Language:

Your body language can convey confidence and assertiveness. Stand tall, make eye contact, and speak clearly and persuasively. Emphasize your arguments with confident and assertive gestures and facial expressions. Consciously adopting assertive body language sends a strong signal that you are confident and in control, which can make you more attractive to others.

## Celebrate Your Uniqueness:

Appreciate your individuality and celebrate what makes you unique. Do not compare yourself to others and focus on your strengths and characteristics. When you accept your uniqueness, you not only increase your self-esteem, but you also attract others who value and are attracted to your authentic self.

Practice self-defense: Confidently share your needs, desires, and limitations with others. Be clear and direct about your expectations, and be assertive when necessary. By defending yourself, you respect yourself and create healthier, more balanced relationships, increasing your attractiveness.

## Take responsibility for your mistakes and successes:

Acknowledge your mistakes and successes and take responsibility for them. If you make a mistake, admit it, learn from it, and take appropriate action to correct it.When you succeed, celebrate it and give yourself credit. Taking responsibility for your actions and results demonstrates trust and authenticity, which makes you more attractive to others.

Embodying confidence and assertiveness is a journey that requires practice, self-reflection, and self-compassion. By embracing these traits, you not only increase your personal attractiveness, you also enjoy healthier relationships, seek meaningful opportunities, and generally lead more fulfilling lives.

# Chapter No. 27

# Finding Balance and Inner Harmony

Finding balance and inner harmony is crucial to increasing attractiveness. When you are balanced and calm within, it radiates outward and draws others to it. Here are some ways you can expand your quest for balance and inner harmony and thereby become more attractive:

## Make Self-Care a Priority:

Make self-care a priority in your life. Take the time to take care of your physical, mental and emotional well-being. Engage in activities that bring you joy, relaxation and rejuvenation. This may include practicing mindfulness or meditation, exercising regularly, getting adequate rest, and participating in activities that encourage self-reflection and self-discovery. Self-care not only promotes inner harmony, but also increases general well-being and attractiveness.

## Cultivating Mindfulness:

Train yourself to be fully present in the present moment and cultivate mindfulness in your daily life. This includes paying attention to your thoughts, emotions, and feelings without judgment. Mindfulness helps you create a deeper connection to yourself and the world around you, promoting inner peace and clarity. When you are focused and present, others are naturally drawn to your calm, grounded energy.

## Establish a Work-Life Balance:

Try to maintain a healthy work-life balance. Set boundaries to make time for relaxation, hobbies, and good relationships. Avoid overworking yourself or neglecting other areas of your life. When you have a balanced approach to work and life, you exude a sense of accomplishment and contentment, which makes you more attractive to others.

## Cultivate Positive Relationships:

Surround yourself with positive and supportive relationships that are uplifting and inspiring. Cultivate connections with people who share similar values and support your personal development. Healthy and meaningful relationships contribute to inner harmony and create an attractive social environment.

## Practice Gratitude:

Cultivate the practice of gratitude by regularly acknowledging and appreciating the positive aspects of your life. This can be accomplished by keeping a journal, expressing gratitude to others, or simply taking a moment each day to reflect on the things you are grateful for. Gratitude draws attention to the present moment and instills a sense of contentment and inner peace that exudes attraction.

## Pursue Personal and Spiritual Growth:

Participate in activities that promote personal and spiritual growth. This may include reading inspirational books, attending a workshop or retreat, or engaging in practices that align with your spiritual beliefs. Striving for growth and expansion on a personal and spiritual level increases your inner harmony and attractiveness.

## Promote a Healthy Lifestyle:

Take care of your physical health by adopting a healthy lifestyle. Eat nutritious foods, exercise regularly and get enough sleep. When you prioritize your physical health, you increase your energy levels, boost your confidence, and radiate vitality, all of which contribute to your overall attractiveness.

## Keep it simple and clutter free:

Simplify your life by organizing your physical space and getting rid of what no longer serves you. Create an environment that promotes calm and clarity. When your physical environment is orderly and free from unnecessary clutter, it reflects a sense of inner harmony and peace and makes you more attractive to others.

## Practice Self-Compassion:

Be kind and gentle to yourself. Give yourself the same compassion and understanding that you would give to a loved one. In times of challenge or setback, show compassion for yourself and acknowledge that you are human and deserve love and forgiveness. Self-compassion promotes inner harmony and self-acceptance, which has a positive effect on your attractiveness.

## Enjoying nature and being outside:

Spend time in nature and connect with nature. Participate in activities such as hiking, walks in the park or just an outdoor picnic. Nature has a calming effect and helps restore inner balance. Staying in nature allows you to recharge your batteries, take a step back and cultivate an inner harmony that attracts others.

## Practice self-reflection and introspection:

Take time for self-reflection and introspection. Journaling, meditating, or having intense conversations with yourself can help you clarify your values, desires, and aspirations. Self-reflection promotes self-confidence and helps you to align your actions with your authentic self, thus promoting inner harmony and attractiveness.

## Accepting and Letting Go of Acceptance:

Train yourself and others to accept yourself and others by accepting imperfections and letting go of judgment and resentment. Acceptance allows you to free yourself from unnecessary burdens and make room for inner peace and harmony. When you exude acceptance, you become more approachable and attractive to others.

## Harness the Power of Boundaries:

Setting and maintaining healthy boundaries is essential to overall well-being and inner harmony. Know your boundaries and learn to say no; if it is necessary. By respecting your boundaries, you protect your energy and create a sense of inner balance. When you respect your needs and boundaries, you not only increase your self-esteem, but also make you more attractive to others who value people with high self-esteem.

## Practice Self-Compassion:

 Treat yourself with kindness and compassion, especially in difficult times. Realize that you are human and allow yourself to make mistakes without being harsh on yourself. Practice self-compassion by speaking kind words of encouragement to yourself and taking care of yourself when you need it most. Self-compassion promotes inner harmony, creates a sense of acceptance and understanding within you, and makes you more attractive to others.

## Cultivate a positive attitude:

 A positive attitude can make a significant difference to your inner harmony and attractiveness. Focus on the good in your life and practice gratitude for the blessings and opportunities that come your way. Challenge negative thoughts and turn them into positive thoughts. By maintaining a positive attitude, you exude optimism and joy, which makes you more attractive to others who are attracted to positive energy.

## Engage in Activities You Enjoy:

Identify activities you enjoy and make them a regular part of your life. Engaging in a hobby, creative pursuit, or activity that sparks your passion nourishes your soul and contributes to your inner harmony. When you engage in activities you enjoy, you radiate a magnetic, vibrant energy that attracts others.

## Practice forgiveness:

 Holding grudges and resentments weighs you down and upsets your inner harmony. Practice forgiveness, both for yourself and for others. Let go of the pain of the past and adopt an attitude of compassion and understanding. Forgiveness frees you from emotional burdens and allows you to move forward with an open heart, making you more attractive to others who appreciate your capacity for compassion and forgiveness.

## Cultivate Healthy Relationships:

Surround yourself with nurturing and supportive relationships that contribute to your inner harmony. Look for friendships and partnerships based on mutual respect, trust, and shared values. Nurture these connections by actively listening, empathizing, and offering support. Healthy relationships provide a sense of belonging and contribute to overall attractiveness.

## Practice mindfulness in your daily activities:

Expand mindfulness beyond formal meditation and incorporate it into your daily activities. Engage in mindful activities, whether it's eating, taking a nature walk, or just having a conversation. By being fully present and aware in every moment, you deepen your connection to yourself and the world around you, fostering the inner peace and harmony that others naturally draw to you.

## Create a Balanced Lifestyle:

 Seek balance in all areas of your life, including work, relationships, hobbies, and personal development. Avoid overstretching in one area and neglecting others. Find ways to balance work and life, prioritize self-care, and make time for meaningful relationships. A balanced lifestyle contributes to inner harmony and demonstrates the ability to successfully move through different aspects of life.

## Seek Support and Advice:

Don't hesitate to ask trusted friends, family, or professionals for help when you need it. Participating in therapy, coaching, or seeking advice from mentors can provide valuable insights and tools for finding inner harmony. When you share your journey with others who can help and guide you, you build resilience and attractiveness.

## Choose flexibility and adaptability:

 Life is full of uncertainties and changes. Flexibility and adaptability allow you to face challenges with grace and maintain inner harmony. Instead of resisting change, approach it with curiosity and an open mind. When you cultivate flexibility and adaptability, you demonstrate your ability to handle life's ups and downs, thereby making you more attractive to others who value resilience and positivity.

Remember that finding inner balance and harmony is an ongoing process. Be patient and kind to yourself as you discover different practices and strategies that resonate with you. When you cultivate inner harmony, you naturally radiate a sense of peace and contentment, which makes you more attractive to others and allows you to live a more fulfilling and balanced life.

# Chapter No. 28

# Celebrating Your Unique Qualities

Celebrating your unique qualities is a great way to increase your attractiveness and boost your confidence. Embracing what sets you apart and emphasizing your individuality allows you to stand out from the crowd and create a magnetic presence. Here are some strategies for developing and acknowledging your unique qualities:

## Introspection:

Take the time to understand yourself better. Think about your strengths and weaknesses, your passions and your values. When you have a clear understanding of who you are, it's easier to appreciate and celebrate your unique qualities.

## Embrace Authenticity:

Be true to yourself. Authenticity is attractive because it shows trust and genuineness. Accept your quirks, interests, and personality traits without worrying about conforming to society's expectations.

## Develop Your Talents:

Identify your talents and invest the time and effort into developing them. Whether you play an instrument, write, paint, or have another skill, honing your talents can make you more interesting and appealing to others.

## Cultivating Confidence:

Confidence is a fundamental aspect of attractiveness. Focus on building your confidence by acknowledging your accomplishments, looking after yourself, setting realistic goals, and challenging yourself to step out of your comfort zone.

## Dress to Express:

Use your own style to express your individuality. Experiment with different mods that reflect your personality, interests, and mood. Dressing in a way that makes you feel comfortable and confident can greatly increase your attractiveness.

## Positive Attitude:

Cultivate a positive attitude and embrace the "I can do this" attitude. Focus on your strengths and focus on development that allows you to learn from challenges and failures. A positive attitude can make you more attractive by exuding optimism and resilience.

## Take Care of Yourself:

In order to increase your attractiveness, it is important to take care of yourself physically, emotionally and spiritually. Engage in activities that make you feel good, such as exercising, eating nutritious meals, getting enough sleep, and pursuing your hobbies and interests.

## Make Meaningful Connections:

Celebrating your unique qualities isn't just about appreciating yourself, it's also about connecting with others. Surround yourself with supportive and like-minded people who appreciate you for who you are. Building meaningful relationships can increase your confidence and attractiveness.

## Participate in continuous development:

learn, explore and broaden your horizons. Be open to new experiences, perspectives and ideas. The constant pursuit of personal growth makes you more interesting and attractive to others.

## Practicing Gratitude:

Developing a sense of gratitude can increase your overall happiness and attractiveness. Appreciate the unique qualities you have and express gratitude for the opportunities and experiences that are presented to you.

## Introspection:

Deepen your understanding of your unique qualities by engaging in activities such as journaling, meditation, or seeking the opinions of trusted friends or mentors. Discover your values, passions and beliefs to better understand what makes you different from others.

## Embrace Authenticity:

Rather than trying to conform to a set pattern, allow yourself to express yourself in all aspects of your life. Share your opinions and points of view openly without fear of being judged. Let your authentic voice shine through conversations and interactions.

## Develop Your Talents:

Take your unique talents and interests to the next level. Attend workshops, courses or seminars to improve your skills. Look for opportunities to demonstrate your skills, e.g. B. by attending local events, joining relevant communities or even starting a passionate project.

## Maintaining Trust:

 Trust is a continuous journey. Practice positive affirmations and imagine yourself embodying confidence in different situations. Regularly take small steps out of your comfort zone, gradually expand it and build resilience.

## Dress to Express:

Use fashion as a creative way to express your personality and unique style. Experiment with different colors, patterns and accessories that reflect your mood and individuality. Consider creating a distinctive style that reflects your personality.

## Positive Attitude:

Develop a gratitude practice by regularly reflecting on the things you value about yourself and your life. Challenge negative self-development and replace it with affirmations that celebrate your unique qualities. Surround yourself with positive influences that uplift and support you.

## Take care of yourself:

Discover different personal care practices that promote your well-being. This may include activities such as bathing, practicing mindfulness or meditation, pursuing hobbies, or seeking professional help when needed. Prioritize self-care to maintain a healthy balance in your life.

## Make meaningful connections:

Participate in activities or join communities that align with your interests and values. Surround yourself with people who value your unique qualities and support your personal development. Nurture these relationships by actively listening, sharing your experiences, and celebrating each other's accomplishments.

## Benefit from continuous development:

Look for opportunities for personal and professional growth. Attend conferences, seminars or webinars in the areas that interest you. Engage in lifelong learning, whether through formal or non-formal education, such as reading books, listening to podcasts, or watching instructional videos.

## Practice Gratitude:

Keep a gratitude journal in which you regularly write down the unique qualities you value in yourself. Express your gratitude for the experiences and lessons that have made you who you are today. Share your appreciation with others and spread the positive attitude.

Remember that celebrating your unique qualities is an ongoing journey. Discover, embrace and constantly develop what makes you unique. By cultivating self-esteem, confidence, and a positive attitude, you can truly show your attractiveness and inspire others to celebrate your uniqueness.

# Chapter No. 29

# Unveiling Your Inner Radiance

Surely! Revealing your inner brilliance is about harnessing your unique qualities and nurturing your inner self. Here are some detailed tips on how to use your inner radiance to become more attractive:

## Self-Reflection:

Take time to reflect on your strengths, values, and goals. Find out what makes you unique and what makes you happy. When you accept your individuality and understand your inner being, you can unlock authenticity.

## Confidence:

Build confidence by acknowledging your accomplishments and strengths. Focus on your positive qualities and remind yourself of them regularly. This inner belief will radiate an attractive aura to others.

## Take Care of Yourself:

To ensure your physical and mental well-being, taking care of yourself is a top priority. Engage in activities that regenerate you, such as exercise, meditation, hobbies, or spending time in nature. When you take care of yourself, you radiate a healthy light.

## Positive Attitude:

Cultivate a positive attitude by practicing gratitude and reformulating negative thoughts. Surround yourself with positive influences and affirmations that will boost your self-confidence. A positive attitude increases your attractiveness and attracts others.

## Emotional Intelligence:

Develop your emotional intelligence by understanding and managing your emotions and empathizing with others. This ability to connect with others on an emotional level fosters deeper and more meaningful relationships.

## Authenticity:

Embrace your true self and let your authenticity shine through. Be honest in your interactions, honestly express your thoughts and feelings, and stay true to your values. Authenticity is very attractive and fosters trust and connection.

## Kindness and Empathy:

Shows kindness and empathy towards others. Be attentive, understanding and supportive. These traits create a positive and caring environment that increases your attractiveness and makes those around you feel valued.

## Lifelong Learning:

Supporting a mindset of continuous development and learning. Engage in intellectual pursuits, discover new interests and challenge yourself. Intellectual curiosity not only makes you more interesting, but also helps you connect with others on a deeper level.

## Cultivate Humor:

Develop your sense of humor and find joy in light-hearted moments. A good sense of humor is attractive and helps create a positive and enjoyable social atmosphere.

## Purpose and Passion:

Pursue your passions and engage in activities that align with your purpose. Purposefulness and passion for what you do add depth and appeal to your personality.

## Practice Self-Compassion:

Treat yourself with kindness and compassion. Accept your imperfections and accept yourself. By being kind to yourself, you radiate inner peace and contentment that others find attractive.

## Cultivate Positive Relationships:

Surround yourself with positive, supportive people who will lift your spirits and inspire you. Foster valuable relationships based on mutual respect and development. Healthy relationships contribute to overall well-being and attractiveness.

## Develop Active Listening Skills:

Practice active listening by giving others your full attention while speaking. Show genuine interest in their thoughts and feelings. By being present and involved, you create a deep connection and make others feel valued.

## Improve Your Communication Skills:

Work on improving your verbal and non-verbal communication skills. Be clear, confident and respectful. Effective communication promotes understanding and strengthens interpersonal bonds.

## Practice Gratitude:

Cultivate a grateful attitude by appreciating the blessings and positive aspects of your life. Express gratitude to others and appreciate their contributions. Gratitude increases your attractiveness by cultivating positive, appreciative energy.

## Develop your talents and skills:

Identify your talents and invest time in developing them. Be it playing an instrument, painting, writing or some other skill, perfecting your skills shows your passion and dedication, which makes you more intriguing and attractive.

## Accepting sensitivity:

Allow yourself to be sensitive and open to others. Share your thoughts, fears and desires authentically. Sensitivity fosters deep connections and shows your willingness to be emotionally available.

## Cultivate a growth mentality:

Accept challenges and see them as opportunities for growth. Focus on learning chess and failing. Growth mentality demonstrates resilience and adaptability, which are attractive traits.

## Practicing mindfulness:

Cultivate mindfulness by being fully present in the present moment. Focus on feelings, thoughts, and emotions without judgment. Mindfulness increases self-esteem, reduces stress and improves overall attractiveness.

## Contribute to the Community:

Participate in acts of kindness and contribute to the welfare of your community. Become a volunteer, support a charity or just help other people in need. Service to others reflects your compassion and generosity, which makes you more attractive.

## Model Positive Body Language:

Pay attention to your body language and make sure it conveys openness, trust and caring. Stand tall, maintain eye contact, and make appropriate, welcoming gestures.

## Developing Emotional Resilience:

Developing emotional resilience by learning to deal with stress, setbacks, and challenges. Build healthy coping mechanisms, ask for help when you need it, and come back stronger. Emotional resilience shows your inner strength and charm.

## Express yourself:

Find creative ways to express yourself, e.g. B. by writing, painting, dancing or singing. Authentic self-expression through art forms allows others to connect with your emotions and experiences.

## Prioritize personal development:

Set personal goals and strive for continuous improvement. Participate in activities that expand your knowledge, skills and experience. Self-development shows ambition and a commitment to becoming the best version of yourself.

## Cultivate a positive attitude:

Maintain a positive attitude even in difficult situations. Focus on solutions instead of dealing with problems. A positive attitude is contagious and attracts people to your optimistic energy.

## Conscious nutrition:

Provide your body with healthy and balanced meals. Watch your eating habits, enjoy every bite and eat mindfully. Taking care of your physical well-being increases your attractiveness.

## Develop Conflict Resolution Skills:

Learn effective methods of conflict resolution and difficult conversations. Practice active listening, empathy and find common ground. The ability to handle conflict with grace and understanding adds to your attractiveness.

## Experience adventure and something new:

Make new experiences, leave your comfort zone and enjoy the adventure. Trying new activities and exploring unfamiliar territory adds excitement and depth to your life and makes you more engaged.

## Practice Self-Reflection and Development:

Regularly engage in self-reflection to assess your thoughts, behaviors, and areas of personal development. Be open to feedback and actively work on improvements. Self-confidence and commitment to personal development are attractive qualities.

## Cultivate a Positive Influence:

Strive to have a positive influence on the world around you. Whether it's through sustainable choices, volunteering, or supporting a good cause, your commitment to creating a better world adds depth and appeal to your character.

Remember that it is a constant journey to reveal your inner brilliance. Check out these detailed tips and adapt them to your unique personality and situation. By taking care of your interior design, you increase its attractiveness and have a positive impact on the environment.

# Chapter No. 30

# Sustaining Your Attractive Self: A Lifelong Journey

## Embrace Self-Acceptance:

Practice self-acceptance by embracing all aspects of yourself, including your flaws and imperfections. Celebrate your uniqueness and learn to love yourself unconditionally. Self-acceptance exudes confidence and attractiveness.

## Lifelong Learning:

Engage in lifelong learning and personal development. Be curious and look for opportunities to expand your knowledge and skills. Participate in workshops, courses or self-study to broaden your horizons. Your commitment to intellectual growth and stimulation makes you fascinating and attractive.

## Cultivate Emotional Intelligence:

Cultivate your emotional intelligence by understanding and effectively managing your emotions. Develop empathy, compassion and self-awareness. Emotional intelligence allows you to connect with others on a deeper level and promotes harmonious relationships.

## Prioritize Self-Reflection:

Regularly engage in self-reflection to evaluate your thoughts, behaviors, and personal development. Take the time to review and evaluate areas for improvement. Self-reflection keeps you grounded and helps you stay attractive through constant self-awareness.

## Maintain Resilience:

Build resilience to recover from setbacks and challenges. Develop coping mechanisms, take care of yourself, and seek help when needed. Resilience increases your attractiveness by showing your strength and ability to overcome adversity.

## Cultivating Authentic Connections:

Focus on making authentic and meaningful connections with others. Cultivate relationships based on trust, respect and mutual support. Genuine connections contribute to overall attractiveness and bring joy and fulfillment to life.

## Practice Mindful Living:

Embrace mindfulness as a way of life. Cultivate present moment awareness, non-judgment and gratitude. Do mindfulness exercises like meditation, deep breathing, or mindful movement.

Mindful living increases your attractiveness by fostering a calm, focused, and balanced presence.

## Promote a Healthy Lifestyle:

Lead a healthy lifestyle by emphasizing exercise, nutritious eating, and getting enough rest. Take care of your body and mind by providing them with food and energy. A healthy lifestyle contributes to your attractiveness by improving your vitality and overall well-being.

## Embodies Positive Values:

Live by a set of positive values that guide your actions and decisions. Be honest, compassionate, and respectful in your dealings with one another. Embedding positive values not only makes you attractive physically, but also morally and ethically.

## Seeking Fulfillment:

Pursue activities and passions that bring you joy and fulfillment. Find meaning and purpose in what you do, be it a career, hobby or volunteer work. Self-actualization increases your attractiveness by exuding a sense of purpose and accomplishment.

## Adaptability and growth mentality:

Promote adaptability and growth mentality. Embrace change, see challenges as opportunities, and stay open to new experiences and perspectives. Adaptability and a growth mentality demonstrate your ability to thrive in different situations, which makes you more attractive.

## Regular Self-Care Rituals:

Develop regular self-care rituals that prioritize well-being. Engage in activities that rejuvenate and recharge you, such as bathing, practicing mindfulness, reading, or pursuing hobbies. Self-care helps you stay attractive by making sure you're always taking care of your physical, emotional, and mental health.

## Cultivate Gratitude:

Practice gratitude as a daily habit. Regularly express your gratitude for the blessings and positive aspects of your life. Gratitude increases your attractiveness by fostering a positive and appreciative worldview that positively impacts your relationships and interactions with others.

## Embrace Your Passions:

Keep discovering and pursuing your passions. Get involved in activities that spark your enthusiasm and bring you joy. When you share your passions and zest for life, you become endearing and attractive to others.

## Practice Active Contribution:

You actively contribute to the world around you. Participate in acts of kindness, support initiatives that align with your values and have a positive impact on your community. Active participation adds depth and charm to your character.

## Cultivate a Growth Mindset:

Adopt a growth mindset that accepts challenges, sees failure as an opportunity to learn, and is committed to continuous improvement. Accept the belief that your skills and intelligence can grow over time. This mindset not only increases your personal growth but also increases your attractiveness as it reflects your drive and resilience.

## Create Strong Boundaries:

Create and maintain healthy boundaries in your relationships and personal life. Learn to say no when necessary and make your well-being a priority. When you respect your boundaries, you convey a message of respect and self-care that makes you more attractive to others.

## Practice Effective Stress Management:

Implement effective stress management techniques to deal with daily pressures and challenges. Find healthy ways to reduce stress such as B. through exercise, meditation, hobbies or time in nature. Effective stress management helps keep you attractive by promoting a calm and balanced demeanor.

## Cultivate your intuition:

Listen to your intuition and trust your inner wisdom. Take the time to connect with your intuition and make decisions that align with your inner guidance. Respecting your intuition will add depth to your character and increase your attractiveness by showing your authenticity.

## Develop Effective Communication Skills:

Constantly work to improve your communication skills. Practice active listening, empathy, and clear expression of thoughts and feelings. Effective communication fosters understanding, deepens connections, and adds to your attractiveness.

## Embrace Diversity and Inclusion:

Cultivate an open and inclusive perspective that values diversity. Appreciate and respect different cultures, beliefs and viewpoints. Accepting diversity increases your attractiveness by showing acceptance and a willingness to learn from others.

## Develop Body Positive Image:

Develop body positive image by emphasizing self-acceptance and self-love. Appreciate and celebrate the unique beauty of your body, regardless of societal norms. A positive body image contributes to your attractiveness by exuding confidence and confidence.

## Practice Active Empathy:

Cultivate active empathy when trying to understand others. perspectives and emotions. Put yourself in their shoes and offer them genuine support and compassion. Active empathy deepens bonds, promotes understanding, and adds warmth to your attraction.

## Embrace Mindful Relationships:

Embrace mindful relationships by being fully present and mindful in your dealings with others. Practice active listening, empathy and emotional availability. Nurturing relationships foster deeper bonds and add to your attractiveness.

## Be Honest:

Live honestly by aligning your actions with your values. Be honest, trustworthy, and accountable for your words and actions. The embodiment of integrity fosters trust and respect and increases your attractiveness in the eyes of others.

## Cultivate a Sense of Adventure:

Feel the spirit of adventure by seeking new experiences, being spontaneous, and stepping out of your comfort zone. Adventures add excitement and vitality to your life, making you more attractive and appealing.

## Develop flexibility and adaptability:

Cultivate flexibility and adaptability in the face of change and uncertainty. Embrace new circumstances, adjust your plans, and find creative solutions. Flexibility and adaptability demonstrate your ability to meet challenges and make you more attractive and resilient.

## Priority Self-Expression:

Express your authentic self through a variety of creative mediums such as art, music, writing or dance. Use self-expression as a way to share your thoughts, feelings, and experiences with others. Self-expression adds depth and richness to your personality and increases your attractiveness.

## Adopt a Positive Attitude:

Cultivate a positive attitude by focusing on the positive side of life, practicing gratitude, and reformulating negative thoughts. A positive attitude is attractive and contagious and creates an uplifting atmosphere in relationships with others.

## Embodies Love and Kindness:

Adopt love and kindness as guiding principles in your relationships with others. Practice compassion, empathy, and the occasional act of kindness. The embodiment of love and kindness not only increases your attractiveness but also helps create a more compassionate and loving world.

Remember that maintaining an attractive appearance is an ongoing journey that requires dedication, self-reflection, and continuous improvement. Follow these step-by-step tips and adapt them to your unique situation and values. By cultivating your inner self and remaining committed to your self-development, you maintain your attractiveness and have a positive impact on the lives of those around you.